Medical Truths Revealed!

Medical Truths Revealed!

Breaking the Misinformation Chain

Find out the Truth about Topics Such As Autism, Alzheimer's, Hormones in Food, BPA Exposure, Artificial Sweeteners, and Much More

MARY ELLEN RENNA, M.D.

SelectBooks, Inc.
New York

Medical Truths Revealed: Breaking the Misinformation Chain

This edition published by SelectBooks, Inc. For information address SelectBooks, Inc., New York, N.Y. 10003.

First Edition

ISBN 978-1-59079-190-5

Library of Congress Cataloging-in-Publication Data
Renna, Mary Ellen.
Medical truths revealed! : breaking the misinformation chain : find out the truth about topics such as autism, Azheimer's, hormones in food, BPA exposure, artificial sweeteners, and much more / Mary Ellen Renna. -- 1st ed.
    p. cm.
Includes bibliographical references.
Summary: "A physician examines science-based studies and medical facts and what she considers to be widespread medical misinformation to arrive at conclusions about controversial health issues"--Provided by publisher.
ISBN 978-1-59079-190-5 (pbk. : alk. paper)
1. Medical misconceptions. 2. Medicine, Popular. I. Title.
R729.9.R46 2008
610--dc22
                        2008034374

Printed in the United States of America

10 9 8 7 6 5 4 3 2 1

Dedicated to my twin brothers, Leonard and Steven,
who were born severely mentally retarded.
Their existence in my life has allowed me to see
the truth about many things, good and bad,
and has given me an immeasurable desire to make
the world a better place for all children.

Contents

Foreword

Over the past decade or so there have been many inaccurate claims made about doctors and modern medicine that perpetuate medical misinformation. This includes the erroneous idea that doctors have cures for diseases that they do not make available to their patients. People who claim this are spreading large amounts of unsubstantiated medical information to the public without any true science to back it up. Since I am a physician, hearing and reading stories about this is particularly irksome. Why would anybody claim that a doctor would not tell a patient that there is a cure or treatment for his or her disease? Most doctors want nothing more than to make their patients well! The spreading of medical misinformation by people who claim they have a "cause" is getting more and more worrisome.

This information is coming from various sources: people trying to make money by selling "natural remedies," naturalists who claim any treatment coming from western medicine is harmful, activists who want to spread "their" word to make changes for the better, and charlatans who take advantage of people in need by making false claims and offers of unsubstantiated treatments. The charlatans come in many different forms, from big industry and small companies to famous people and book sellers. The sellers of herbal supplements, cold and flu "remedies," and "colonic cleansers," as well as many others, can also fall into this category. Is the public supposed to accept someone's word about important health topics without proof or an evidence base?

I believe the public wants to know all sides of medical topics. They do not want to hear uninformed opinions, but instead want to hear hard data about such controversial topics as environmental toxins, hormones in food, vaccines and autism, prevention of Alzheimer's, the dangers of sugar and cell phones, and the benefits of alternative medicine. For those of you who want to hear what science is saying about many of these topics, this book is for you!

Introduction

This book was inspired by my great desire to reveal the truth about the many medical issues discussed in the 21st century. These issues are often written about by non-medical people who spread information that can be incorrect, misleading, sensationalized, or just complete lies; a better word for this is medical "propaganda." Propaganda is the giving of information to people only for the benefit of the person who is *giving out* the information. This is in direct contradiction to education that is the giving of information for the benefit of the person *receiving* the information.

The plethora of medical propaganda has pushed this misinformation chain to the point of endangering our families' and our own health. We are bombarded with information from books, television, newspapers, magazine articles, and the Internet. It can be difficult to sift through all this information from the media to pick out the real science from junk science. As a pediatrician to thousands of patients, I have many parents who turn to me for answers to their questions about many of these health topics.

The use of the Internet has exponentially increased the delivery of information, but at what price? Anyone can start a web site to make false and unsubstantiated claims, and thousands of people now have web sites spreading their propaganda! This is one of the main reasons there is so much false information that can be extremely dangerous. If a website looks good and seems to have been written by professionals, many people assume the information is correct. All of us need to look at information on the Internet with a discerning eye.

I have had the fortune to appear on television to discuss various medical topics with non-medical people. I have talked about lead in toys with parent health advocates and the relationship between obesity and soft drinks in schools, but the most interesting and eye opening topics are the ones that deal with vaccine issues. I have learned some important lessons when trying to talk with individuals who are involved in fighting to change vaccination policies or trying to "educate" the public about vaccines. One of the lessons is that when people have an "agenda," they have no desire to hear what someone with a different opinion, even with medical expertise to back it up, has to say. Another lesson I have learned is that most of these people, whether from a lack of training or a lack of desire, have either false information obtained from the Internet or incomplete knowledge of the subject matter. They tend to be the types of people who want to change medical policies despite their lack of medical training. Nothing is more frustrating than trying to EDUCATE individuals when they are not interested in hearing the medical truth being revealed to them!

I have compiled many of the most controversial questions about medical issues and put together cohesive answers based on medical experience and research. The answers may seem surprising, especially if we have information ingrained in us that is not necessarily based on scientific facts but is perpetuated through the misinformation chain. This erroneous knowledge is passed on simply because we fail to continually ask questions and seek answers. If we feel comfortable with an answer to a problem, the tendency is to look no further. But the answers can change from decade to decade depending on the amount of research going on in any particular field. If we are satisfied with an answer and then stop asking questions, we may never find the truth. For those people who want to look further, the answers can be disappointing as well as reassuring or surprising.

The questions in this book are not always easily answered. There is usually more than one way to look at a problem. Many times it can be like looking into a prism; the information scatters in many different directions. Often people try to simplify an answer, and this is a dangerous way to think. One highly emotional topic is autism and its causes. This is a perfect example of how we may simplify a very complicated issue. For example, at the present time there is no known *single* cause of autism; however, there are people who believe that a change in diet can "cure" autism. Autism is most likely caused by many factors. If we believe the people who are making these claims about diet without any medical studies to substantiate them, and we assume that food allergies play a major part in the etiology of autism, many parents will be given false hope. This may deter them from using much needed medically backed therapies as they try unsubstantiated "treatment" in the hope of a cure.

It is also important to identify people who participate in research that may "have an agenda." People who work for agencies designed to protect our health, or people involved in research, *may* have a view point that is driven by extreme emotion, power, or money. Some people work for companies funding research projects; others may have financial or emotional ties to the company without being an employee of the company. If these people cannot be objective, their information may be unreliable. Without objectivity, data cannot be interpreted properly.

Big companies may benefit or be harmed by the results of a particular research project. Some of the studies I reviewed to help answer the questions posed in this book were done by researchers who have connections to companies that either funded the studies or companies that would be affected by the results. The possibility of research bias always exists, but when money and big industry are involved, a sharp, suspicious eye is needed to review the studies.

I do not have any agenda, other than to help find the truth and to do what is best for our children. I am tired of seeing "practitioners of health" trying to sell *their* agendas to vulnerable people. As the medical misinformation chain is growing in leaps and bounds, their job of selling junk medicine becomes easier and easier. The "practitioners of health," as I like to call them, are either people who do not have any credentials, or those who have limited medical credentials but insist on making medical claims without substantial research to back up their claims. They then try to "sell" the information to the public. This can be in many forms. For example, a non-medical person may write a book claiming to have "cures" for diseases that doctors are keeping from the public, an activist can make claims while attempting to change medical policies, or a company can claim to have supplements for sale claiming they help to stop the aging process. This can also be in the form of "practitioners of health" advising against getting the flu shot because it is "more dangerous than contracting the actual flu virus"! Vulnerable people, persuaded by these claims, come in all forms. People are especially vulnerable when they become parents because the fear of possible harm to their children clouds good judgment. But we all can be vulnerable to listening to those who talk a good game in spite of what 21st century science tells us.

I want to find the answers, wherever they may lead me. I am not selling a product or an ideal. I am merely trying to disperse science-backed information. Some people may not want to hear the answers to the questions in this book. They have already come to conclusions based on what they have heard on television or read in a magazine and are already convinced that they have THE answer. A parent in my practice asked me about hormones in milk. When I told her the results of my research, she very quickly said, "I don't agree with that." I asked what she knew about hormones and milk and where she received her information. I reminded her that she was not reading any medical studies on this topic, that she knew little about the digestive system of humans and how hormones work, but was instead listening to a newscaster on TV or reading an article written by a journalist. I had to explain to a very intelligent woman, that she was getting her information from the misinformation chain. She immediately understood what I was talking about and was willing to take what I said as the truth.

The chapters in this book will not be the end of the story. They are merely a stepping stone to finding an answer that is based on research and professional experience and NOT from the misinformation chain.

Who Are the "Practitioners of Health"?

As I have stated, these are people who have limited or no knowledge of medicine or disease, yet attempt to treat all sorts of ailments with their "protocols" or make medical accusations without research to back up their claims. Complementary and alternative medicine practices (CAM) are becoming more popular as people look to find answers outside of western medicine. Complementary therapies are used as an adjuvant to mainstream therapies in the form of helping to control symptoms or enhance well being. Some of the complementary therapies have proven to be safe and effective and have become integrated into mainstream medicine. Alternative therapies, on the other hand, are offered as alternative treatments to mainstream medicine. Using unproven therapies as a replacement for conventional treatment is usually a dangerous scenario, although there are some alternative therapies outside of conventional medicine that may have some efficacy, especially in the form of benign nutrient supplementation.

However, there are two important factors to consider when using CAM therapy. The first is to make sure you are working with a reputable CAM practitioner, and the second is to make sure your conventionally trained physician knows what alternative therapy you may use. It is difficult for pediatricians to condone alternative treatments, in the form of herbal remedies, because little data exists to prove that these therapies work, especially for children. Because there is no standardization of herbal remedies, children (adults also) could be exposed to dangerous contaminants that cause severe reactions. It is much safer to use FDA regulated and approved therapies because we know what we are getting when we take an FDA regulated medication, we know what we are treating, and we are aware of the side effects.

People with cancer are particularly vulnerable to alternatives outside of standard medicine. If you were diagnosed with cancer, how many of you reading this book would be willing to go to an alternative health professional rather than seek out a trained physician to guide you to the best surgeon and oncology doctors? The problem occurs when the limits of Western medicine are reached and people feel the need to look somewhere else. I empathize greatly with these people because it only makes sense to try everything in an attempt to be healed. The problems I encounter are with the endless medical imposters who claim they want to help, use lots of non-researched backed treatment, and make a lot of money doing it.

There are many practitioners who are willing to take advantage of a person's adverse situation to make a great deal of money. I am certainly *not* trying to say that all people who are not conventionally trained in medicine are charlatans. I want to make people more aware of what to look for when they are seeking medical advice outside the realm of conventional medicine and to know when the situation is hurting rather than helping them.

Thank goodness I have not been in a situation where my children or family were not responding or being treated successfully with Western medicine. But for the past two decades I have seen other people search for unconventional help. Most of the time their experience was unsuccessful and costly.

A very dear friend of mine gave me insight into the minds of people who are in desperate need of medical help after trying all the conventional medical avenues. She had been suffering from severe back pain for years, had multiple back surgeries, and was on a host of pain killers. Unfortunately, she was still in pain and the pain killers made her depressed and tired, a bad situation for a young woman. A friend told her about a wonderful "therapist" who helped her with her back pain by using a special massage technique. So my friend had to try it. She showed up at the house of an older couple where the gentleman was going to be the one to treat her. She was told to get completely undressed and to lie down on his massage table. He started to massage her with the usual massage technique. There was nothing unusual at first, but as he continued to massage her, she realized he was massaging every inch of her body, which was **not** the standard massage technique. This was being done while the man's wife was in the kitchen cooking. This sounded like something out of a movie with a bad ending.

When she told me the story I could not believe it and asked her if she was going crazy. Her response was a very poignant and insightful one. She said, "When you are in pain, emotional or physical, you'll try anything to get help and if someone tells you that drinking cat urine will help you, you'll drink the cat urine." Being in a situation of pain, fear, anxiety, or illness can lead people to go against their better judgment and try a "remedy" that will cure them, alleviate pain, and end their suffering. I have since seen many people on the brink of "drinking cat urine" to get help for their child. I was glad to be there to offer help to them. I am being dramatic here, but some of the remedies that have been given to my patients were not only shockingly useless but potentially harmful.

Of course there are good complementary therapies that are used in conjunction with conventional medicine. They include mental health support and development, yoga, acupuncture, and massage. These are generally very helpful and may also be great stress relievers, which we know from experience can help to decrease symptoms of disease.

There are some parents in my practice who are suspicious of conventional medicine but still take their children to me for illnesses and yearly evaluations. I remember one parent who sought out the opinion of an "alternative doctor" for her son's illness. Her son was a healthy child but had come down with a sore throat and temperature. The alternative doctor evaluated my patient, diagnosed him with strep throat *without a throat culture* and sold the mother an herbal "cure." The total for the visit was over $300.00. The mother was concerned about the diagnosis of strep and decided to come to see me to elucidate things. She explained the scenario to me, and now it was my job to help her son. I examined her son, did a throat culture, and diagnosed him with a viral sore throat. I then explained to the mother that no doctor can diagnose strep throat without a throat culture (unless the patient has scarlet fever) and if he did think her son had a strep infection it is unacceptable *not* to give him antibiotic treatment. The danger of untreated strep throat includes rheumatic fever, kidney disease, throat abscess, and even death, all of which should not occur with the proper use of antibiotics. The mother responded that I "was confusing her" and she did not know who to believe! Now I must tell you that having a medical degree as well as practicing pediatric medicine for the past twenty years makes me capable of diagnosing the cause of a simple sore throat in a child. It was also bothersome to know that this irresponsible "doctor" received over $300.00 for his services. I tried to explain to the mother that she was being taken advantage of because of her desire to avoid antibiotics. In this particular circumstance, the "doctor" pretended to make a diagnosis of strep throat to sell her some ridiculous product that she believed would help her son while at the same time avert the use of antibiotics.

Parents of children diagnosed with autism are particularly vulnerable to people claiming they have the next new cure for autistic children. I have many patients in my practice who have been diagnosed with some form of developmental delay, and of course the parents would do anything to help their child. My overall feeling about complementary therapies for autism is that if it does not harm the child, I am willing to try most things. But I will never give a family false hope. If they hear that a milk-free diet is helping children with autism, I will not stop them from a dietary change. I do tell them not to get their hopes up. There are doctors popping up all over the place claiming they can help children with autism. The people who are helping autistic children the most are the wonderful, caring team of therapists who spend their days teaching these children. The neurologists and developmental specialists are also instrumental in the care of these children. They do not make claims about the cause of autism, such as food allergies, metal poisoning, or an environmental toxemia, but instead perform a medically targeted work-up that may include blood work or imaging procedures. The doctors to be wary of are the ones who require hundreds of dollars for a consultation, then more money to do a non-medically targeted work-up on blood or urine to try to find an abnormal lab value or an environmental toxin. They then ask for additional money for the treatments they want to sell you. It is very likely that one day we will identify many environmental toxins that may cause autism when a developing fetus is exposed to them; the genetic material of a person will probably be what determines how much and which toxins will increase susceptibility to a future diagnosis of autism. For now it is better to avoid putting you and your child through unproven testing or treatment unless you are part of an academic study run by a reputable institution.

Section I

Vaccines, Autism and Environmental Toxins

The increase in the number of children being diagnosed with autism has caused a frenzy of theories from many sources. Unfortunately, some theories that gain huge audiences are not based on medical knowledge and come from biased sources. Because there are few persons on this earth who are not concerned about children and the possible harm from external insults, bringing up key words such as autism, toxins, or cancer during a discussion about inoculations from vaccines is certain to get everyone's attention.

The next few chapters will deal with the topic of vaccines and autism, vaccines in general, flu vaccine, the possible ways to prevent autism, and environmental toxins and the role they may or not play in generating illness.

The first chapter deals with autism and vaccines. I have researched this area very carefully. I have been on the "front lines" of giving out the vaccines and have seen almost all the possible side effects from the vaccines, new and old. I will talk about the results of my research as well as twenty years of experience in giving out the vaccines during these changing trends.

I will also talk about some possible ways to actually decrease the risk of having an autistic child. There is much to be learned about autism, but I have applied the information that we know now to actions that may translate into decreased risk.

1

Vaccines and Autism ...
Does A Link Exist?

A day does not go by in my practice without a parent asking me questions such as, "Is it safe to give immunizations?" or "Are you positive nothing bad will happen from this vaccine?" or "She is not going to become autistic, right?" Autism is more widely diagnosed now than it was forty years ago; one of the main reasons is that the criteria for diagnosis has changed over time and more children can be included in the diagnosis than in the past. Along with an increase in the diagnosis of autism there has been a decrease in the number of children who are diagnosed with mental retardation (a diagnosis that is based on IQ). It is possible that children in the past who were diagnosed as mentally retarded are now being diagnosed as autistic.

The rise in diagnosis of autism along with the media attention given to an article by Andrew Wakefield in the British journal *The Lancet* in 1998 that made an MMR–autism link a scientific possibility, ignited an unusual amount of fear surrounding vaccinations.

Let's take a look at some of the vaccines and the diseases they are protecting us from before taking a look at the possibility of a vaccine–autism link.

The early days of the vaccine era brought about great sighs of relief from the public. At last we had the ability to protect ourselves and our children from the devastating effects of diseases like polio, tetanus, diphtheria, whooping cough, and smallpox. These diseases brought about disability, disfigurement, or death.

13

They were very real diseases that people encountered. Parents saw what happened to the child next door who developed polio; suddenly, a vivacious child running around in the grass could no longer walk. Communities were shut down and pools closed to stop the spread of virus during an outbreak of polio. Pictures of children in the iron lung were a reality. They also witnessed first-hand what a disease like diphtheria could do to a person, and whooping cough was a common occurrence. When these diseases were running rampant and people were afraid of being stricken, the development of a vaccine was nothing short of a miracle. Few people worried about side effects from vaccines; they cared only to be protected from the devastating diseases that they saw first-hand. The devastation and fear for their children during outbreaks of polio, measles, diphtheria, and whooping cough was far worse than fear of any side effect from vaccine.

The oldest vaccine on record was one developed for the small-pox virus. When smallpox swept through communities it killed up to 30% of the people affected. The 18th century brought about a vaccine for smallpox. Even then some people were skeptics. Benjamin Franklin was not an advocate of the vaccine and did not want to vaccinate his family. Unfortunately, he lived to regret his decision when his son died from smallpox in 1736. He lamented his mistake and begged other parents not to do what he had done.

Diphtheria vaccine was introduced into wide use in the 1940s. In the early 1900s diphtheria was the leading cause of death in children between the ages of 4–10 years. Pertussis, also known as whooping cough, is a continued worldwide health threat. Before the introduction of the vaccine, virtually everyone was exposed to whooping cough and 1 in 750 babies died before the age of one from whooping cough. In 2004 the WHO estimated that there were 300,000 deaths from whooping cough despite vaccine efforts.

In the 21st century we have eradicated smallpox, polio is on its way out, death from whooping cough has been drastically reduced, and the annoying and occasionally fatal chickenpox is a rarity—all because of vaccines. Because many of these diseases are not a real-ity to parents, some are hesitant to vaccinate their children. For them the threat of disease is not real enough to counteract the fear of a possible reaction to a vaccine. Not being actively threatened by disease is, of course, a wonderful luxury, but what most people are forgetting is that vaccines have brought us to this point.

The children who are getting vaccinated take the minimal risk of a vaccine reaction in order to receive protection from a disease. They are also making a huge contribution to the protection of children who are *not* being vaccinated. This is a phenomenon called "herd immunity." When most people are vaccinated for a particular disease, the illness is much less likely to take hold in a community, thereby protecting the non-vaccinated individuals. This herd immunity, along with good health care, has been the reason that many diseases have been kept to a minimum or wiped out completely. However, as more and more parents choose not to vaccinate their children, any one of these diseases will be able to take hold in a community.

An example of the breakdown of vaccination use that resulted in disease resurgence came about in the early 1990s. After the fall of the Soviet Union in the 1990s, the health care system was disrupted and immunizations fell to the wayside. A diphtheria epidemic occurred that affected tens of thousands of people and killed almost 5,000 people between 1990–1993. Unfortunately, people need to be reminded how quickly these diseases can take hold and wipe out communities without vaccine protection.

Measles is one of the deadliest diseases in history and has been feared for centuries. When epidemics hit, they wiped out thousands of people at a time. The virus's only host are humans, and despite vaccine efforts it is still around to do damage. The main reason this virus has such staying power is its extreme contagiousness and its ability to be carried by healthy people to cause disease. In the 1960s, before the introduction of the vaccine, one person every 15 seconds died from measles worldwide! After the introduction of the vaccine, the incidence of measles dropped by 98% in the United States. It has been estimated that over the first 20 years of vaccine use, 52 million cases of measles were prevented; this meant that over 17,000 persons did not end up mentally retarded (a complication from measles encephalitis), and approximately 200,000 people did not die from the disease.

Measles, unfortunately, is still around. As the trend to move away from giving the MMR vaccination continues, more children will be put at risk for measles. A resurgence of measles virus occurs when the vaccination rates drop. This has been proven time and time again. One example of this in the United States was in 1990 when the measles vaccination rate dropped to a low of one in two children. The population became vulnerable to the virus, and, sure enough, 55,000 cases of measles were reported between 1989 and 1991 with over 120 deaths. There are many more examples of the measles virus taking hold in a poorly immunized community and killing people; it is very clear that when measles immunity rates fall, the disease comes in and does harm. We need to stop learning the same lesson over and over again, and we must vaccinate our children against this deadly virus. Until all evidence of measles is wiped from the face of the earth, our children and grandchildren will be at risk.

The media has a tremendous impact on society. Since the reporting of the 1998 study by Andrew Wakefield and colleagues stating a possible autism and MMR link, the number of children receiving MMR vaccine has decreased. The news media reported on the results of the study without being able to properly interpret the validity of the work. The only message parents were hearing was that MMR vaccine can cause autism. The majority of parents have probably never heard of someone coming down with measles, mumps, or rubella. Since these diseases were not a legitimate threat in the minds of parents, the fear of the vaccination overtook the good sense of some parents who opted not to give the MMR to their children. The Wakefield study that set off this chain of events has since been vastly criticized. Some of the authors have retracted their data. Unfortunately, the damage had already been done from this study and resulted in public wariness of the MMR vaccine. The medical community has since published many studies looking at vaccines and autism.

The first two years of life are when the majority of vaccinations are given. This is the time when language and communication skills are developing. This is also the time when child development that is going awry is recognized. So how do we separate the possibility that vaccines bring on autism as we try hard to protect our children by vaccinating them in their first years? Since we know that millions of lives have been saved because of vaccinations, there would seem to be no doubt that everyone should want and have the luxury of being protected from vaccine-preventable disease. But in today's society many regard the diseases that we are vaccinated for as only a "theoretical risk," and this misinformation leads people to think that any vaccine reaction, no matter how mild, may be unreasonable and dangerous. This way of thinking contributed to the sensationalizing of the Wakefield study, and prompted many parents to start asking themselves whether the "risk" of vaccination was worth it.

Let's take a more careful look at the most current literature on possible vaccine-autism links. Research studies have looked at thimerosal exposure and autism, timing of vaccination and autism, and persistent viral infection from live vaccinations and autism.

Thimerosal is the mercury preservative that was and is still used in vaccines. It is found in multi-dose vials of influenza and immunizations that are used in third-world countries. The major vaccines given in the U.S. no longer contain thimerosal because the American Academy of Pediatrics lobbied to have it removed from vaccines. The academy was concerned that babies were cumulatively getting too much mercury from all the vaccines given to children. It was subsequently shown that babies who had been fully vaccinated with thimerosal-containing vaccines had mercury levels below the EPA acceptable limits, but there are no plans to put thimerosal back into vaccines in the US.

Mercury is a known neurotoxin, but ethyl mercury, the form of mercury in the vaccines, is eliminated quickly from the body and has a more difficult time crossing into the brain than the toxic methyl mercury found in our environment. The question of whether or not thimerosal was the cause of the apparent increase in autism has been a focus of many studies. To this date studies have not found a causal link between thimerosal exposure and autism. To put this matter into perspective, we can look at autism rates since the removal of thimerosal in vaccines. Babies receiving vaccines prior to the removal of thimerosal received approximately

200 micrograms (mcg) of mercury during the first two years of life. Currently, a baby is exposed to less than 3 micrograms (mcg) of mercury from vaccines, but as the mercury exposure from vaccines has been decreasing, the rates of diagnosis of autism is still on the upward trend! A recent study in the *New England Journal of Medicine* evaluated thimerosal exposure in a group of 7–10 year olds. They calculated the amount of thimerosal exposure for each child and then subjected them to a battery of neuropsychological tests. The study did not reveal any significant difference in 42 neuropsychological areas within varying levels of thimerosal exposure.

There were many studies on this subject and the overall consensus is clear: there is no causal association between autism and thimerosal in vaccines. The World Health Organization still uses thimerosal in millions of vaccines because no association with autism has ever been shown.

When the 1998 study by Andrew Wakefield suggested MMR was causing autism, it set off a frenzy of studies to address the accusation. MMR vaccine is given for the first time between 12 months and 18 months, the same time that developmental problems are usually recognized. It seemed as if the timing of the vaccine and the diagnosis of autism were linked causally. This is not the case. The linkage is merely in timing only. A new study to come out of England *was looking for an association* between measles and autism spectrum disorders, the hypothesis being that the measles virus persists in children who are affected adversely by the vaccine.

Let me diverge to explain how live vaccines work to protect us. The MMR is a live attenuated virus vaccine. The injection of live but weakened virus into a child is the way immunity is achieved with the MMR vaccine (as well as some other vaccines). The weakened but live virus injection elicits an immune response that can be used later *if* the real virus comes along. The virus is eventually cleared from the blood with the end result of antibody production for future use. This is very similar to what happens when we get infected with any virus, but the vaccine virus strain is in a much weaker state. This new controlled study I mentioned above was attempting to prove that children who received the MMR vaccine and developed autism did so because the body was unable to clear the vaccine virus from the body with a resultant persistence of the infection in children who later were diagnosed with autism. The study *did not* find any difference in measles antibody or persistence of measles virus in children diagnosed with autism versus the control group. Another study looked at the use of the MMR vaccine in England (the Wakefield study came out of England). MMR vaccine use began there in 1988. Researchers looked at rates of autism in children born in London between the years 1979–1998. The diagnosis of autism in the time period before and after use of the MMR vaccine did not reveal any change in the rate of diagnosis. Study after study has failed to uncover any association between MMR and autism.

The development of vaccines has been by far the greatest health contribution to society, but to say it has been smooth sailing would not be true. There has been a history of vaccine disasters. The use of a contaminated BCG vaccine, a vaccine used to help prevent tuberculosis, killed 72 infants in 1929–1930. In the early days of the polio vaccine, a batch of insufficiently attenuated virus was used that infected 120,000 children; 51 children were paralyzed and 5 children died. We learn from these disasters and do not make the same mistake twice.

In the mid-1990s the DPT vaccine was reformulated because of concerns about complications from the vaccine. The new acellular DTaP vaccine has a better safety profile and is just as immunogenic as the old vaccine. Vaccine safety is a high priority for everyone involved, and I can say that the vaccines given in the United States are of the highest quality with minimal risk of side effects. A vaccine must undergo phase I, II and III human trials that can take up to ten years before the FDA will consider it for licensing. There is continued post-licensure surveillance to watch for side effects while the vaccine is given to millions of people. The FDA also requires *each* lot of vaccine to be tested before it can be released for use.

I have been giving vaccinations to children for over twenty years. The only unfortunate scenarios from this experience were when parents refused to vaccinate, and the child subsequently became infected with the vaccine-preventable disease. Thank goodness there was not any long term disability from the disease infection in these cases.

A worry that I hear quite often is the fear of "bombarding" the immune system with multiple vaccines given at one time. Before a vaccine can become licensed, data must be shown on the safety and effectiveness of the vaccine. The data also looks at the antibody response when multiple vaccines are given together. This is done to make sure there is no interference from other vaccines in the amount of protective antibodies being made for a given immunization. Not every vaccine is tested with every other vaccine. However, there are guidelines that the pediatric practitioner must follow that allow certain vaccines to be given together without reactions.

One argument that is being thrown around is that the young immune system cannot handle the load of antigens (foreign substances) being given at one time, causing a subsequent abnormal brain response that leads to autism.

The injecting of foreign antigens into babies should not, and is not, taken lightly by medical professionals. Is it possible that somehow the vaccine or substances in the vaccine is causing some autoimmune phenomenon with a subsequent deterioration in brain development or myelinization? This theory does not hold water because if there were an autoimmune event with abnormal myelinization in the brain, an MRI would likely pick up the abnormalities. The results of brain MRIs in autistic children are usually normal.

Could it be possible that the multiple injections given at one time causes a short-lived depression in the immune system that allows a live virus vaccine to persist in the blood? As I have said, this theory has been disproved because researchers have never isolated vaccine virus from immunized children with autism.

Could it be that the number of vaccines given at one time is too much for the baby's body to handle? Many parents ask me this exact question. My response usually is a question. I ask them what they mean by "too much to handle." When I ask this question of a parent I am not trying to be glib because I would never belittle a parent's worry. I merely need to get more information to understand what his or her main concern is. Are there unknown effects of giving multiple vaccines at one time? Are there unknown effects of giving vaccines one at a time? My answer to both questions is, "We have been giving multiple vaccines since the development of the DPT vaccine in the 1940s and have seen many side effects, but I am sure that autism is not one of them. I also am sure that the risks of not vaccinating far outweigh any possible risk of vaccinating."

There is no connection between autism and vaccinations. Study after study has proven this, yet the trend toward limiting immunizations continues, putting our children at risk for disease and even death from vaccine-preventable disease. To continually banter the vaccine and autism relationship when the vaccines have not changed significantly is a waste of precious time, energy and money. It is time to look in other places to find the causes of autism, in particular the endless area of environmental exposures during pregnancy.

Every parent should feel good about giving all the recommended vaccinations to their child!

.

2

The Flu Vaccine in the 21st Century

Caring for sick children is always a challenge and often parents and patients ask how I manage to stay healthy and avoid getting sick. My response is always the same: "Of course I get sick." It is impossible to avoid the viruses from children who are coughing in your face or wiping mucous from their noses and then touching your face. A pediatrician's only hope is that we have already seen the virus and made antibodies to protect ourselves.

The flu virus is a different story. This nasty little virus has adapted itself so that every few years it changes just a little bit, rendering the antibodies made in our body in the past less effective. Even worse, every few decades the virus may change dramatically, rendering our antibodies completely useless for defense and causing worldwide pandemics. A perfect example of this is the 1918–1919 flu pandemic that killed 20 million people around the world. Other examples are the Asian flu of 1957 that killed 70,000 Americans and the Hong Kong flu of 1968 that killed 34,000 Americans. To really put death from flu or complications from flu into perspective, the fact is that it was the sixth leading cause of death in 1990. The only way to be protected from the flu without locking yourself inside for the winter is to get the flu vaccine.

I see hundreds of patients with viral illnesses each winter season, and I am very careful to wash my hands and to remind the children to wash their hands frequently to help prevent viral spread. Another important way to prevent viral spread is to cover a cough with an elbow rather than the hand to minimize aerosol droplets flying through the air. While I have been relatively successful in avoiding contact with the flu virus, there have been two times in my practice when I have been in the direct line of fire of mucous flying out of a nose or mouth of a child with the flu. (My office uses a rapid flu test so we can accurately diagnose the flu). When I say I was in the direct line of fire, I mean the mucous fell directly on my lips and tongue. The mucous was teeming with flu virus because the mucous from both the children tested positive for the flu. The parent of one of these patients was so horrified that she called me multiple times during the next week to make sure I was okay. She talks about it to this day, and we still laugh out loud when remembering the incident. Now, of course, I can blame only myself for being a mouth breather and allowing the offending mucous to have access into my mouth. Both times that I was exposed to a heavy burden of influenza virus directly into my oral mucosa, I had already received the flu vaccine. Needless to say, I did not get the flu and my patients recovered from their flu.

I have not always been so fortunate, because I have indeed been unlucky enough to get the flu. It was a year when vaccine was in short supply, and I decided to forego the shot for that year. What a huge mistake that was. That year was the only time I ever had the flu, and to top it off, I came down with a horrible pneumonia that I would most likely have died from had it not been for antibiotics. I ended up missing two weeks of work and felt weak for a month. Needless to say, I have not skipped a year since then.

My testament to the vaccine should not be enough to convince you that the flu vaccine is needed and can save lives, but I wanted to give you a personal story. I will talk about the history and statistics of the flu vaccine and then dispel a common myth about the vaccine. Hopefully, you will come away with a better understanding of the flu and how dangerous this virus is to humans.

The burden of influenza has been written about since the time of Hippocrates. Ancient cultures were better shielded from flu epidemics because the virus requires crowds of humans for the virus to take hold and spread from person to person. The small towns and lack of mass transportation in the past caused the virus to die out relatively quickly so that major flu epidemics were not as problematic as other highly transmissible diseases. As the world became more populated with people living closer together and using mass transportation, the virus could spread to many people very quickly, causing epidemics.

The onset of the flu virus is usually abrupt and causes severe body aches, fever, runny nose and cough. I had a little girl come in to my office complaining, "My hair hurts." She, of course, had the flu, because almost nothing else makes you feel so sick. It is not uncommon for the children who have the flu to ask me if they are going to die. It is heart-breaking to watch children suffer from this terrible virus and even more so to hear them worry about dying because they feel so horrible.

The virus replicates in the respiratory epithelium from your nose down to the smallest parts of your lungs. It destroys this protective lining and causes swelling and sometimes bleeding and scarring. The virus itself can cause a deadly pneumonia that is usually refractory to treatment. Pneumonia, along with other bacterial infections, is frequent after infection with the flu virus and is a common cause of death after influenza infection.

Over the past several years the flu has claimed the lives of 20–150 children per year under the age of 18 years old. The vaccines that are available include a trivalent dead virus vaccine and an intranasal live virus vaccine. Since the live intranasal virus vaccine is new and can be used only in individuals between 2 and 50 years old, I will keep the discussion and the data results limited to the inactivated flu shot. (I am a huge fan of the intranasal vaccine and the early data coming out shows that it may be even more effective than the inactivated shot.)

A common misconception is that the flu shot gives people the flu. This is impossible since the vaccine uses parts of the virus's outer coat and is not live. When the vaccine is injected into the body, it stimulates antibody production to the viral strains in the vaccine. When we get an actual viral infection, not only is the virus making us feel sick, but our immune system fighting off the infection also makes us feel sick. This is why some people may not feel great after receiving the vaccine.

Each year the vaccine consists of three strains of flu. The three strains to be used in the vaccine are picked the prior season. Based on the prevalence of each strain the previous year, it is decided which strains will be included in the vaccine for the oncoming flu season. There have been times when the predictions were off and the major circulating strains were not included in the vaccine. This is because it is impossible to accurately predict which strains will take hold when the flu hits.

Any time anyone gets a vaccine there may be side effects. They include mild allergic reactions, sore arms, muscle aches, fever and, very rarely, severe allergic reactions. As I have said already, many of the reactions are due to the immune system mounting the proper response for future fight against the real flu virus. These are almost always very minor reactions and a lot less severe than actually getting infected with the flu virus.

In 1976 the swine flu vaccine was associated with an increased risk of Guillain Barré syndrome (GBS). This is a rare neurologic disorder that causes a reversible paralysis and is known to be associated with other viral or bacterial illnesses. No one knows why that particular flu vaccine triggered GBS in certain people, but since then the association of GBS with the flu vaccine is *below* the baseline rate of 1–2 per 100,000 people.

Unfortunately, the "practitioners of health" (the groups of people with limited or NO medical training who give people medical advice) attempt to put fear into the minds of the public by exaggerating or holding onto ideas about complications from the swine flu vaccine of 28 years ago. They also do this by making claims that the vaccine is more dangerous than getting the flu, or that the preservative thimerosal causes autism, or that "toxins" are left in the body after the vaccine. I have read a book written by a non-medical person claiming that the vaccine has done nothing to help deter death from the flu! The misinformation chain is at work and I want to set the record straight for those of you who doubt the vaccine's efficacy.

The elderly, who are most at risk for death from the flu virus, make up about 90% of all deaths from flu each year. The only exception to this statistic is during pandemics, which mainly claim the lives of healthy young adults. The death statistics vary each year. From 1973–1995 the numbers of deaths in the U.S. varied between 20,000 to over 40,000 deaths, with most occurring in the greater than 65 year age group, and to a lesser extent in babies younger than 6 months who are too young to receive the vaccine.

There is a decreasing efficacy of the vaccine in the people that need it most—the elderly. After the age of 70 the efficacy of the vaccine is reduced because of the declining immune system of the elderly; they do not mount a good immune response to the vaccine. Over the age of 80 years the vaccine may not have any effect in preventing death from the flu. More research needs to be done to address this area, but the best-case scenario is to target the population that is most likely to spread the virus. Children play a big part in the transmission of the flu virus in a community. Making the flu vaccine mandatory for any child attending day care or school would help to limit the spread of the flu each year. The new recommendation is to vaccinate all children 6 months to 18 years of age. If we all did our part in trying to prevent the flu, we would see a dramatic decrease in the morbidity and mortality of the elderly, as well as in young babies.

Using *conservative* numbers, vaccine efficacy in the young can range from 50–70% if the strains in the vaccine are matched correctly with the circulating strains. There are some years where the vaccine is much less effective; some studies showed that only 25% of vaccine recipients were protected from the flu due to a mismatch of the strains. However, even with a mismatch, the vaccine is still beneficial. For all the non-believers out there, let's do a little math.

The vaccine rates for high-risk adults are between 30–50% and the rates for high risk children are even lower, falling between 10%–30%. If 90% of all flu deaths are in the high-risk category of people over 65 years, that means between 18,000–36,000 people over the age of 65 die each year from flu. For argument's sake, we will assume that the efficacy of the vaccine in elderly individuals is extremely low. Since there is a waning of the immune system in the elderly, the vaccine does not make protective antibodies as effectively as it does in younger individuals. In this population if we use a vaccine efficacy of 10% and take the vaccine rate to be 30% for this population, 12,600–25,200 of the elderly people did not get vaccinated and 1,260–2,520 did not need to die from the flu. The 2000–4000 individuals left over are mainly young babies, children and young adults. If we use a 50% *overall* efficacy for the flu vaccine (which is an extremely low percent) in the younger population and assume that only 10% of this population *was* vaccinated, that means that 900–1,800 individuals died that could have been protected with the flu vaccine. That is a lot of people who did not need to die.

It is always important to ask questions and challenge research by doing more studies. However it is dangerous to take your own opinion about the flu vaccine to persuade a high-risk individual not to take the vaccine. Some "practitioners of health" who have dissuaded high risk individuals from receiving the flu vaccine must live with the possibility that some of these people may have died from the flu.

3

Is It Possible to Reduce My Risk of Having An Autistic Child?

Why are more children being diagnosed with autism than ever before? Are there better diagnostic criteria or is the rate of children with autism really on the rise? Some people argue that children are not born with autism but develop it after an insulting event after birth. Other people feel that autism is a combination of genetic potential triggered by an unknown event before or after birth. This chapter is designed to answer these questions and to come up with some sensible science-backed ways that MIGHT reduce the chances of having a child with autism.

Autism is generally defined by impairments in three areas: Reciprocal social interaction, abnormal verbal and nonverbal communication, and restrictive, repetitive, or obsessive behavior. These behaviors need to be present before the age of three in order for the diagnosis of autism to be made.

It appears that the rate of autism is on the rise. But are we really seeing an increased incidence in this disorder or are there other factors at play? There aren't any laboratory or radiologic tests that can diagnose autism so we rely on the *Diagnosis and Statistical Manual of Mental Disorders, Fourth Edition, Text Revised (DSM IV TR)* for specific criteria for medical personnel to use when evaluating children. Over the past 25 years the diagnostic criteria for autism have changed with each edition of the manual. The broadening of the criteria has included children in the diagnosis that in past years have not been included. This

29

artificially raises the incidence rates because more children are now being diagnosed, not necessarily due to an increase in the disorder but because we accept more children into the diagnosis.

Another reason the rates may appear elevated is because children are starting to be diagnosed at a younger age. Children diagnosed at a younger age will again artificially raise the rate of autism because at any given time more children are "diagnosed" with the disorder.

With that being said, studies have looked at the prevalence of autism over time while taking into account these confounding variables. The end result is that autism is unfortunately on the rise with no end in sight. This is not good news. As a pediatrician I can say that I see more children present with signs of autism now than when I first started to practice pediatrics in 1990.

Why is this happening? At the present time there is no SINGLE cause of autism identified. Researchers have seen a chromosomal aberration on all but three chromosomes in children diagnosed with autism, but no single genetic abnormality has been identified. Genetics does seem to be involved in the development of autism. The probability of a sibling being diagnosed with autism is increased by 5% compared to the general population, and the probability of an identical twin being diagnosed with autism is increased by 60–90%! That implicates a genetic predisposition. The many therapists and physicians that have been helping autistic children will agree that autism does indeed have a genetic component. I started to notice this many years ago in my private practice, when often, families would have more than one child with developmental problems. It has been only recently that science is starting to back this theory.

Genes are not the complete story. Many professionals feel that a combination of genes and some external insult results in the development of autism, but the external insult remains a mystery.

The possibilities of heavy metals, infections, pesticides, pollution, immunizations, hormones, artificial insemination, and even *in vitro* fertilization have been suspected as possible insults resulting in autism. An increased risk of autism occurs in some genetic diseases such as tuberous sclerosis, phenylketonuria, and some viral infections that happen *in utero*. I will not talk about diseases that cannot be prevented or avoided, but instead I will stick to medical issues surrounding autism where it may be possible to alter risk factors.

Before I start to talk about the possible ways to decrease autism risk, I must re-emphasize that there is absolutely *no* association between autism and immunizations. It is my privilege to give children life-saving vaccinations each day, and competent pediatricians, trained in the specialization of caring for children, would not continue to do something that is harmful to patients.

Study after study has without a doubt exonerated any immunization as a cause of autism. Thimerosal (the ethyl mercury containing preservative) in the vaccines has also been exonerated; many studies have backed this statement. Thimerosal has been used as a vaccine preservative since the 1930s. In the 1990s it was noted that the cumulative amount of *ethyl* mercury children received from the immunizations was above the acceptable level of exposure that the EPA set for *methyl* mercury exposure. I am distinguishing between the two forms of mercury because there was no data on ethyl mercury toxicity from vaccines, outside of allergic reactions, so all the data used to decide to change the vaccines came from methyl mercury data. The methyl mercury is the environmental mercury that is very toxic, crosses the blood brain barrier and stays in the body over long periods of time. Depending on the type of vaccine used and the weight of the baby, it was possible that some babies were getting higher levels of allowable mercury (based on data from toxic methyl mercury) but in the form of ethyl mercury. As a precautionary measure the CDC, The Public Health Service and The American Academy of Pediatrics recommended that vaccine manufacturers remove thimerosal from vaccines.

Almost every vaccine that is now given to children in the United States is thimerosal free. The total ethyl mercury exposure for babies under 6 months born in the past few years is virtually zero. Unfortunately, the rate of autism is still increasing despite eliminating ethyl mercury from the vaccines. This data alone helps confirm that thimerosal in the vaccines was not one of the causes of autism.

Let's move on to possibilities that have some data to back them up.

Mercury is a known neurotoxin that humans are still being exposed to on a regular basis. The term "mad as a hatter" came about from the chronic mercury exposure that occurred in the hat industry many years ago. The hat workers toiled in poorly ventilated rooms for long hours. Because mercury was used to make the felt that was used in hat production, the workers making the hats underwent chronic inhalational exposure to mercury. Over time the workers unfortunately developed behavioral changes and other central nervous system changes.

The most common form of mercury exposure today is a form of organic mercury that occurs because of environmental contamination from industry waste. The seas are contaminated with *methyl* mercury which subsequently contaminates sea creatures. The most common form of mercury exposure in humans occurs with fish consumption, especially fish that are predatory and feed on other fish. We have seen the devastating effects of mercury toxicity in fetuses after the Mimimata Bay contamination in Japan. The bay was heavily contaminated with industrial methyl mercury and the fish were subsequently exposed. The fish were consumed by pre-pregnant and pregnant women with devastating effects on their offspring. The mothers did not display any signs of mercury toxicity. However, the children were born with deafness, blindness, seizures, inability to talk, limb deformities, and mental retardation. Because the developing fetus is much more sensitive to mercury exposure than the mothers, the mercury crosses the placenta and the blood brain barrier to cause devastating effects on the baby while leaving minimal toxic symptoms in the mother.

Although this type of exposure is from chronic high-dose exposure, in today's society we are more at risk for chronic low-dose exposure. This chronic low-dose exposure in utero has revealed an association with deficits in language, attention, and memory in children. There is no proof that mercury exposure causes autism, but because it is such an obvious neurotoxin for fetuses, it is best to avoid mercury exposure when pregnant or thinking about becoming pregnant.

For women thinking about becoming pregnant or who are already pregnant, this means to avoid eating fish that are long-lived, for example, such fish as tuna, swordfish, shark, tilefish, bass, and king mackerel. Other short-lived fish contain much lower levels of mercury and can be consumed in moderation during pregnancy.

Alcohol is a know teratogen. Teratogens are substances that disrupt gene expression and may therefore cause a malformation or a series of malformations. The "fetal alcohol syndrome" occurs in pregnancies when alcohol is consumed during pregnancy. The exact amount of alcohol that causes a problem is not known, so the recommendation is to completely avoid alcohol exposure during pregnancy. The more alcohol consumed, the greater the probability of developing the syndrome. Fetal alcohol syndrome has many features, including delayed development and mental deficiency. The degree of neurologic issues can range from severe mental retardation to mild developmental delays. Since alcohol is known to disrupt brain development, it is crucial to stay away from alcohol while pregnant. At the present time there isn't any data proving alcohol causes autism per se, but its effects on the developing brain can be devastating.

Cigarette smoking during pregnancy is associated with a four-fold increase in the likelihood of delivering an abnormally small or premature baby. The more cigarettes smoked, the greater the possibility of a devastating outcome. The more premature a baby is, the greater the chance is that there will be lifelong problems like learning disabilities, mental retardation, or cerebral palsy. If you smoke, it is wise to quit before you get pregnant and make sure you avoid cigarette smoke throughout the pregnancy.

Congenital rubella syndrome is the result of a mother contracting rubella (German measles) during pregnancy. Women who contract rubella during the early weeks of pregnancy are likely to give birth to babies with severe problems. Cataracts, deafness, heart defects, immune defects, and hormonal problems are just some of the abnormalities that occur as a result of congenital rubella. Up to 30% of babies with congenital rubella syndrome are diagnosed with autism. *This is a completely preventable form of autism.* It is extremely important for all women to be completely immunized against rubella. It is still a common infectious disease in developing countries and can put a non- immunized woman at great risk when pregnant. Congenital rubella infection should not be a cause of autism because we have long had the vaccine to protect us. No women should be giving birth to a baby with congenital rubella syndrome. Get vaccinated!

Pesticides are another area that needs to be looked into. The environment is loaded with pesticide residues. Practically all humans have traces of pesticides in their bodies. The ability to detect pesticides and pesticide metabolites in human tissue has become so sophisticated that chemists can detect pesticides in amounts that measure in the parts per trillion! With this new sophisticated analysis technique, studies have been done that find pesticide residues everywhere inside the human body. It is almost impossible to avoid exposure to pesticides. One study looked at babies born in NYC and found six different organophosphate pesticides in their first stool! Pesticides have been found in the amniotic fluid of mothers undergoing routine amniocentesis. Pesticides were even found in the breast milk of native Alaskan women living an indigenous lifestyle.

How does this fit into the story of how you can decrease your risk of giving birth to an autistic child? It is not easy to find one chemical that may or may not be linked to developing autism because we are exposed to so many other chemicals on a daily basis. However, there are studies that have looked at particular pesticide exposure during gestation with poor neurological outcomes.

Studies have shown that children born to fathers who were pesticide applicators had an increased risk of having neurologic developmental impairment that included autism spectrum disorders and ADHD.

Chlorpyrifus (an organophosphate pesticide used widely in agriculture) and its metabolites have been shown to interfere with the developing brain of experimental animals. A herbicide commonly used, 2,4-dichlorophenoxyacetic acid and its metabolites have been found in the milk of lactating animals. These substances altered chemical reactions in the developing animal pups being breast fed, and as a result caused behavior changes like apathy, reduced social interaction, and repetitive movements in the experimental animal. These behavioral changes in the lab animal sound all too much like some behavior changes seen in autistic children.

A recent study out of California may show the closest link between autism and the damaging results of pesticide exposure during gestation. The study identified a relationship to autism of "pesticide drift" exposure during pregnancy. The closer a pregnant woman lived to a field delivering pesticides, the greater was the likelihood of her giving birth to an autistic child. The farther away a pregnant woman lived from a farm spraying pesticides, the less likely was she to deliver a baby that was diagnosed with autism. This study is the beginning of proof that certain pesticides in the environment are a toxic insult that can cause autism in genetically susceptible individuals. The main pesticides in this study were dicofol and endosulfan.

If a woman is considering getting pregnant and lives near a farm that uses pesticides (within 500m), I would recommend finding out which pesticides are used. I would then try to stay far away from the site before and during pregnancy.

There is nothing that can guarantee delivering a healthy baby, nor is there anything that can guarantee delivering a child free of any neurological or behavior issues. There are, however, things that every woman should take to increase the odds of making a physically and neurologically healthy baby.

Every woman considering getting pregnant should not smoke cigarettes before or during pregnancy. I would strongly recommend that every woman of childbearing age (or everyone for that matter) be completely immunized to decrease the risk of acquiring a vaccine-preventable disease, especially one that has as association with autism, such as rubella. There are other viral infectious diseases that have a link to developmental issues, but since there is no vaccine to prevent them, I have not discussed them here.

Also, every woman who is considering getting pregnant must stay away from alcohol. At the present time there is no documented acceptable limit of alcohol intake during pregnancy, so alcohol should be avoided altogether. Likewise, any woman considering getting pregnant should also avoid organic mercury exposure at all costs. The main exposure occurs through eating fish, so it is beneficial to keep large predatory fish like swordfish, tilefish, shark, tuna, and king mackerel out of your diet before you get pregnant (for at least six months) and while you are pregnant. Do not avoid fish all together while you are pregnant because of the tremendous health benefits of omega 3 fatty acids to you and the baby. The last recommendation I would make is to eat organic foods while you are pregnant and avoid any undue pesticide exposure in your daily life. If eating organic is too expensive or just not feasible, try to stay away from the fresh foods that tend to absorb the most manmade pesticides, such as peaches (the highest by far of all foods), spinach, apples, pears, and squash. There are plenty of other good fruits and vegetables that can fill the void while you are pregnant.

As I said before, nothing can guarantee that you do not give birth to a child with autism, but following the above recommendations will help to increase the odds of delivering a healthy baby!

Organic Foods: The Use of Hormones, Antibiotics, and Pesticides in Our Food

The "go green" movement has gained momentum as it attempts to curtail an endless array of problems that modern society has wrought upon us. Many theories, solutions, and speculations have come from the green movement, while its members push the benefits of organic foods and warn humans of the potential harm that pesticide usage is having on our environment.

Organic farming has increased considerably over the past decade, making the availability of organic foods ever-present in the supermarkets. The increased cost of producing organic foods is passed onto the consumer, but the price for going green may not only be hitting our wallets.

Hormones and antibiotics used in farming have become another issue for the population to worry about. As hormones found in milk and meats are making headlines, we need to understand what the risks may or may not be in regard to their consumption. We have the same issues raised about the use of antibiotics in agriculture because many fear its potential to cause more devastation to our health. The following chapters will look at the facts and give some solid answers.

Our environment is becoming more and more filled with industry by-products and chemical pollutants. These chemical pollutants are found in our food, water and even the air we breathe. What is the damage to humans that is occurring from these contaminants in our environment? Is there a price we are paying for having all the luxuries modern society has brought to us? Is the use of potentially toxic pesticides justified? There are too many questions to answer, but I will touch on the most prevalent topics in this area.

4

Organic Foods: Are They Really Better for Us?

A very common question that parents ask about is the use of organic foods for their families. There are many factors that are involved in deciding whether organic foods are better for consumption, but first we need to understand what constitutes organic foods. The USDA certifies foods as organic if the food has been grown without the use of *pesticides, hormones, or antibiotics.*

To answer the question of whether eating organic foods is better than eating non-organic foods, we need to look at the WHOLE picture of pesticides and food availability. The misinformation chain starts when questions are not dissected properly and the answers become over-simplified. We need to take into account all the issues that arise from growing produce organically versus non-organically as we look at the question from many different angles. If we come up with a rational, science-based conclusion that organic fruits and vegetables will have a substantially positive impact on the individual, we then need to be sure that it is not at the expense of the population as a whole.

There are many people who subscribe to the belief that organic foods are the only foods that should be consumed. At first glance this seems to be an obviously intelligent way to live one's life. Who could argue with not wanting to ingest plant foods that have had a myriad of chemicals sprayed into the dirt they grew from or onto the plants themselves? It seems to make perfect sense not to eat animals that have ingested pesticides on a daily basis. It may also seem obvious that avoiding foods from animals that are given hormones is a good idea. Our body makes all the hormones we need. Since we don't need any extra hormones why eat it in our foods? The use of antibiotics in the agricultural industry is also a cause for concern. Antibiotic usage in animals has increased over the past years and the effects have already been seen with resistant bacteria popping up all over the place. Unnecessary exposure to antibiotics can cause more harm than good. So what effect is the use of antibiotics in agriculture having on humans?

In this chapter I will concentrate on the chemicals in organic fruits and vegetables. Hormones and antibiotics are used mainly in animals and the question of hormones and antibiotics will be addressed in later chapters.

The questions that need to be answered before I can tell if organic foods provide a significantly increased health advantage over non-organic foods are:

1. Does the possible pesticide residue that may be ingested in fruits and vegetables pose a risk that can be measured over time?

2. Is there any negative effect that can be attributed to eating organic foods?

3. Do organic foods contain more nutrients?

4. Does the possible pesticide residue that may be ingested in fruits and vegetables pose a health risk that can be measured over time?

A pesticide is any substance used to deter the growth of weeds, molds, mildew, fungi, or plant-destroying insects. The EPA (Environmental Protection Agency) has set limits on how much pesticide is allowed to be used on plants grown for consumer ingestion. Limits have also been set on allowable *pesticide residues*. Pesticide residue is the amount of a specified chemical substance in any agricultural commodity that is left on the plants as a result of pesticide use. This is different from contaminants like mercury. Contaminants are substances that are not intentionally added to foods and can occur in organic or non-organic foods.

The EPA evaluates many avenues of exposures to chemicals before it determines whether a chemical is safe for widespread use. It evaluates acute exposure toxicities such as skin burns, mucous membrane irritation, and neurotoxicity. It also analyses chronic exposures to chemicals to evaluate reproductive toxicity, mutagenic potential, carcinogenic potential, or hormonal disruption potential. The level of allowable pesticide residue in food is based mainly on experiments done on lab animals (mainly rodents); there is also some human data that has been used, but much less than with experiments using rodents. The endpoints that are used are mainly the carcinogenic and mutagenic potential of the pesticide being tested. After determining the safety of a chemical, the EPA sets limits on allowable exposures by extrapolating the data to humans. The acceptable daily intake (ADI) for each of the major pesticides is determined by the data. The ADI is the level of pesticide that a human can ingest on a daily basis without any *appreciable* risk over a lifetime of exposure. The level set by the EPA is usually much lower than the lowest dose found to have an effect on lab animals. Once the EPA sets the amount of pesticide use allowable on a particular crop, the amounts must be adhered to by the farmers.

Before we can tell if the ingestion of manmade pesticide residues is causing disease, we have to take a good look at our environment to see what else may be contributing to our disease burden. Ingesting pesticide residues in foods is not the only way we are exposed to pesticides. It may be impossible to separate disease burden caused by pesticide residue in food from other toxic environmental exposures. Many of us use pesticides in our homes on a routine basis. We use mold killers to clean our bathrooms, antibacterial sprays and wipes for our kitchens, and insecticide sprays for pest control. We are exposed to some form of chemical in almost every aspect of everyday life.

Picture a typical day of many Americans. We arise from a bed that has a chemically dry-cleaned bed spread, and detergent-cleaned and fabric-softened sheets that lie on top of a chemically treated wood-framed bed. We walk on stain-resistant carpeting to the bathroom. Most likely the bathroom has been cleaned with some sort of cleanser containing pesticides. After a shower we put on deodorant and use some hairspray. Then we go to the kitchen to make a cup of coffee, heat up the gas stove, cook eggs in a Teflon pan, toast bread, and sit on a chemically treated chair before we head off to work. Getting into the car we drive off to work. We stop to get another cup of coffee in a Styrofoam container and pick up a plastic water bottle to drink from during the day. Depending on the nature of our job we may be exposed to many more chemicals at work. Out at lunch we ingest thousands of natural pesticides and chemicals in our meal. After work a trip to the barber shop, hair salon, or nail salon provides a plethora of chemical exposure. Then it is time to go home to our perfectly manicured lawns; the use of various weed killers, growth promoters, and pesticides has assisted in keeping the lawn looking fine. Inside the house ants or termites may have existed, but with the use of pesticides they are eradicated. At the end of the day we have a nice fish dinner and put the kids to bed in their flame retardant pajamas!

There are of course many more ways we are exposed to chemicals on a daily basis. It would be a difficult task to fully describe the amounts and types of chemical exposure that we experience in a single day.

I am merely trying to give you a glimpse of the ways we are exposed to manmade chemicals during a typical day.

While the present estimate is that 250,000 manmade chemicals are used in our environment, it is also estimated that about 10,000 *natural* chemicals from plants are ingested from our foods. This means that humans are exposed to a significantly larger amount of plant-made chemicals on a daily basis than to any manmade chemicals. Interestingly, 99.9% of the chemical exposures in humans are from the ingestion of natural plant-made chemicals!

These plant-made chemicals are part of the natural defense system that enables plants to fend off predators and to help protect the plant against environmental damage. There are thousands of natural chemicals made by plants to help ensure their survival. Many of these chemicals are good for humans; when they are thought to promote good health they are known as phytonutrients. The phytonutrients that plants produce to protect them from environmental damage can have the same function for humans when ingested. Some act as antioxidants that fend off the dangers of free radicals. Other types of phytonutrients help kill cancer cells and others absorb cholesterol to help maintain heart health. We are only at the tip of the iceberg when it comes to understanding the benefits of these phytonutrients.

Some of these natural plant chemicals, however, may be harmful to humans. These are chemicals from the plant-manufactured defense system known as plant pesticides. Most plants are not edible because they contain large quantities of these natural pesticides that are toxic to humans. Not only are they inedible, but they can be deadly if eaten. As a matter of fact, one of the most common poisonings in children occurs from accidental plant ingestion.

It has been estimated that humans ingest 1500 milligrams of natural plant pesticides in a day, but only 0.09 milligrams of manmade pesticides per day. Unfortunately the manmade pesticides we ingest in foods are the same ones that have caused increased cancer levels in agricultural workers as well as increased birth defects in their children.

What does this mean in terms of the average consumer? Almost all our food has pesticide residues on them. According to the EPA 73% of fresh fruits and vegetables contain pesticide residues (only 61% of processed foods contain residues of pesticides!) The foods that have been identified as having the largest toxicity index (most pesticide residues) are fresh peaches (identified as the highest by far among many fruits and vegetables tested), apples, grapes, spinach, pears, and squash. Foods that have the least amount of pesticide residues are milk, orange juice, broccoli, bananas, canned peaches and canned or frozen corn.

And here is the main point: lab studies done on plant manufactured pesticides reveal that they are as toxic as manmade pesticides! Of the natural plant-made pesticides studied, 50% of them were rodent carcinogens, which is roughly the same percent as the synthetic pesticides.

If we only take into account the amount of chemicals ingested from each category (manmade versus plant made) it would seem that natural pesticide ingestion presents more of a health hazard than synthetic pesticide residue ingestion. Fortunately, in this case, the data from rodent testing is not always a good indicator of toxicity. Usually, the dose of the chemical used for testing in the rodent is much greater than the average amount ingested by humans; this means that rodent carcinogenicity testing does not necessarily translate into human carcinogenicity. *Small doses of many chemicals can be tolerated well, but in larger doses they can be deadly.*

How do we use this information to our advantage? As I have said, we are exposed to thousands of chemicals on any given day and it is very difficult to try to decipher whether manmade pesticide residues in foods are the sole cause of a specific health problem.

Eating small amounts of EPA approved pesticides does not cause the same effects as other types of large exposures to toxins (this data does not pertain to the developing fetus). A small exposure from approved pesticides has no little or toxic effects if we are in good health with a normal detoxification system—which includes our gastrointestinal system, liver and kidneys. This may be difficult to understand so let me give you an example of what I mean. Commonly used over-the-counter medications, such as antihistamines and decongestants, are relatively benign medications when taken at proper doses. Parents have been using these medications on their children for years without any thought of possible harm. However, at higher levels of exposure caused by improper dosing or intentional overdose, these relatively harmless medications can become deadly! It comes down to how much the body can handle at a given time. If our detoxification system is overloaded, the most innocuous chemical may become deadly.

The reverse is also true; a toxic chemical can be innocuous at low-dose exposure. This is a very important concept to understand because the synthetic pesticide residue ingestion from food is very small. This makes the toxicity virtually nil in a healthy person.

It can be argued that it is better not to expose the human body to any toxins; why stress the body into having to expend energy absorbing vitamins and minerals to get rid of the chemicals we should not be eating anyway? What if our detoxification system is not working well because of poor nutrition or illness? I could continue to ask theoretical questions about synthetic pesticide exposure in the foods we ingest, but as I have tried to point out, we are exposed to so many chemicals in our environment, as well as natural pesticides in foods, that it is virtually impossible to avoid "toxin" exposure. The ingestion of manmade pesticide residues is dwarfed by the amount of natural plant-made pesticides humans ingest each day. More importantly, we have lab data that has shown some of the natural plant-made pesticides to be as toxic as synthetic pesticides. Since there is no data looking at the effect of eating the natural plant pesticides in the organically produced foods, we can't comment on the health effect this may have on the individual. Now you can get an idea of how tricky it is to answer a question without looking at all the details.

What we can say is at the present time, there are no documented studies linking manmade pesticide residue ingestion in foods to any illness or cancer.

Is there any negative effect that can be attributed to eating organic foods?

The answer to this question may seem very obvious, but first we need to know how plants survive without the help of manmade chemicals.

I already talked about plant pesticides and phytonutrients that plants manufacture. Another class of plant-made chemicals is called anti-nutrients. These are plant-derived chemicals that directly interfere with the absorption of essential nutrients in humans. For example, phytates found in grains and seeds interfere with the absorption of minerals, while oxalates in spinach, rhubarb and tomatoes interfere with calcium, iron and zinc absorption.

We eat plenty of these anti-nutrients in fruits and vegetables, but there is no real difference in the amount ingested when comparing organic and non–organic foods. It is good news to find out that the plant foods that humans ingest on a regular basis have many more phytonutrients (plant nutrients) than anti-nutrients.

Foods that are produced organically contain more natural pesticides than foods produced with manmade pesticides. Organically-produced foods need to make more natural pesticides to fend off predators since they are not getting the "advantage" of the synthetic pesticides. As I said, there is no data looking at the effect of eating more plant pesticides in the organically-produced foods. We know from tests based on rodents that the plant-made pesticides seem to be as "carcinogenic" as synthetic pesticides, but not all of the plant-manufactured pesticides have been tested.

Since there is no data on the effect of ingesting plant pesticides and organically-produced fruits and vegetables contain more plant-manufactured pesticides, I cannot conclusively say that there are more detrimental effects attributed to eating organic fruits and vegetables as compared to those produced conventionally.

It seems clear that maintaining health is a balance between nutrients, anti-nutrients and pesticides (natural or synthetic) in the fruits and vegetables that we eat.

Are organic foods more nutritious than conventional fruits and vegetables?

There are more nutrients in most organic foods as compared to the same food produced non-organically. Pesticides reduce the amount of vitamin C, beta carotene and other B vitamins thereby reducing the amount available in conventionally grown foods. Organic foods also have lower levels of detrimental heavy metals like mercury and lead, and higher levels of helpful minerals like selenium and calcium.

When manmade pesticides are used in crop production, the plants do not have to work as hard to defend against predators so they make less natural-defense chemicals. This means they make less of the good phytonutrients but also less of the plant pesticides. When foods are produced organically, they need to make more of the defense chemicals to protect them from environmental dangers. Thus they make more phytonutrients and more plant pesticides.

Organically produced foods have been shown to contain as much as 40% more phytonutrients compared to conventionally produced crops.

It is safe to say that organic fruits and vegetables have higher levels of certain nutrients than conventionally produced fruits and vegetables. They also contain less harmful contaminants. It is possible that the increased nutrient intake along with a decreased contaminant exposure will have a positive health impact on the individual but this can't be said with certainty. The small dose of contaminants may have absolutely no impact on the individual; the same goes for the increase in some nutrients.

To sum it all up: It is prudent to eat a *variety* of fruits and vegetables on a regular basis to minimize pesticide exposure and deter nutrition associated disease. To categorically state that eating organic fruits and vegetables will have a substantial impact on disease burden is not backed up by scientific data. If you have the luxury of choosing organic foods, pick the organic foods, that when produced conventionally absorb the most manmade pesticides (such as fresh peaches, apples, spinach). There are times in a woman's life where I feel it is beneficial to eat organic. The developing fetus is particularly vulnerable to manmade pesticide toxicity (there IS data to substantiate this), so my recommendation for pregnant women is to only eat organic foods to minimize all possible risk to the baby.

If it comes down to eating non-organic fruits and vegetables versus not eating fruits and vegetables at all, the data is very clear. The risk of diseases due to lack of fruit and vegetable intake is far greater than any possible risk of ingesting pesticide residues in fruits and vegetables, whether manmade or plant-made (except during pregnancy and lactation).

5

Are There Hormones in Milk that Will Affect Me or My Child?

Another way to ask that question is: What effect does bovine somatotropin (cow growth hormone) have on the milk from cows who received the hormone?

The word "hormone" evokes many emotions in humans. For many of us these emotions are usually negative ones. The emotional reaction elicited when we hear the word "hormone" is most likely caused by the misinformation chain, erroneous information passed on from one person to another until it appears as if the information is scientifically founded. The truth is that all animals need hormones to stay alive. Hormones are chemical messengers that perform vital functions for living beings. Animals cannot exist without hormones. We have seen the devastating effects of type I diabetes that are caused by the lack of insulin production. With the use of recombinant hormone, the life of millions of diabetics has been saved.

Unfortunately, humans have found a way to abuse certain hormones. We have all heard about the damage that hormones can cause when used outside the realm of medicine. For example, anabolic steroid use in athletes has been known to cause a myriad of future health problems. Even some hormones used in medical settings can have very dangerous side effects when used for long periods of time. But more importantly, the use of hormones in humans improves quality of life, cures some diseases, and saves lives.

Hormones are used in agriculture not to save animal lives but to increase the production of a commodity. Whether the commodity is milk or meat, hormones help to increase overall production. We will take a look at the use of hormones in animals and the possible effects they may have on humans.

Bovine somatotropin is the naturally occurring hormone in cows that is involved in the production of milk. Recombinant bovine somatotropin (rbST) is a genetically engineered version of the hormone that is given to cows to increase milk production. Use of rbST in cows has generated much fear, controversy and conjecture. Let us take a look at some facts on rbST.

Recombinant bovine somatotropin is used in cows to increase milk production. Most cows increase their milk production by about 10-15% after rbST is used. The hormone is given by injection before the cow's milk dries up after giving birth. The recombinant hormone has been found safe to use by the JECFA (the joint UN food and agriculture organization and the WHO expert committee on food additives), the FDA and many other regulatory agencies. I will not take their word on the safety of its use so let's probe a little deeper.

There are other hormonal effects that occur in the cow from the use of rbST. The use of this hormone causes increased levels of IGF-1 (insulin like growth factor) in the cows. Insulin-like growth factor is found naturally in humans as well as in cows. The IGF-1 is the hormone that ultimately produces the effects of growth hormone to promote growth. The levels of IGF-1 in the milk of treated cows are slightly higher than non-treated cows. But it is interesting that the levels of growth hormone in the milk from cows not treated with growth hormone are the same as the levels found in treated cows. What does this mean? Does this information translate into trouble for humans consuming milk from cows given rbST?

The use of rbST in cows may translate into higher levels of IGF-1 in consumer used milk. Some studies in humans have shown a link to cancer and increased serum levels of IGF-1. It can be assumed that *if* levels of IGF-1 are increased in humans from ingestion of milk from hormonally treated cows, we may be at increased risk for some cancers.

It is always dangerous to make assumptions without looking at all the data. We still do not have enough information to answer the question of whether consumption of milk from cows that received rbST will cause harm to humans. As I stated, milk from cows treated with growth hormone has the same levels of growth hormone as cows *not* treated with growth hormone. As a matter of fact, we have been drinking bovine somatotropin since cow milk was first used for human consumption, which is about 10,000 years ago. The hormone has always been present in cow's milk as a naturally-occurring hormone! Not only have we not seen any detrimental effects from drinking cow's milk over the past centuries, but instead we have seen the use of cow's milk increase the chances of survival for many babies after they were weaned from the breast. Since it appears that drinking cow's milk (with hormones) has been a boost to our survival, why should we be concerned now? The story is not quiet complete.

We know that the level of insulin-like growth factor IGF-1 has been found to be slightly elevated in the blood and milk of cows treated with rbST. The elevated levels of IGF-1 in hormonally-treated cows' milk has been shown to be within the range of "acceptable limits." Unfortunately, there have been some studies linking elevated serum levels of IGF-1 in women with certain cancers (more studies need to be done to further elucidate any possible connection with IGF-1 and cancer in humans). The human body does makes its own IGF-1, but the question here is whether increased amounts of IGF-1 in consumed cow's milk translates into *increased* levels in the blood of humans.

First of all, much of the IGF-1 is destroyed during the heat processing of milk. Secondly, IGF-1 and rbST are both proteins that are destroyed when ingested by humans. This means that even if we drink the hormone in higher than normal levels, it will not have any effect on us because we destroy it in our digestive tracks. Even if we were **injected** with bovine growth hormone, it would not have any effect on us because it does not work as a hormone in humans.

Finally, let us take a look at the milk quality of hormonally-treated cows compared to cows not treated with growth hormone.

The nutrition content of milk from treated verses non-treated cows is virtually the same. Protein, vitamin, mineral, sugar, and fatty acid content are not significantly changed. One of the differences that has been noted in treated milk is that there is a higher content of unsaturated fats. So, if anything, the milk is a healthier product!

There is still active research in this area, but at the present time there does not seem to be any undue risk from drinking milk from cows given rbST. The milk has no known hormonal effect on humans.

6

What Hormones Are Used in Meat and Are They Dangerous to Consumers?

Growth hormone is a protein hormone used in dairy cows to increase milk production, but there are also six steroid hormones used in cattle to promote growth and increase the yield of meat. They are used through an implant to deliver a certain amount of chemical over time. The amount of hormone in the implant is the smallest amount to give the animal the most growth. These hormones are not used in chickens, turkeys, or pigs. The hormones used are estradiol, progesterone, and testosterone, which are the same hormones that are manufactured in humans. Also used are the synthetically made hormones trenbolone acetate, melengestrol acetate, and zeranol, which mimic the action of testosterone, progesterone and estradiol respectively. It should be noted that trenbolone has anabolic activity several fold greater than testosterone, and melengestrol has 30 times more progesterone activity than natural progesterone.

The steroid hormones are different from the bovine somatotropin discussed in the previous chapter because steroid hormones can be absorbed when taken orally, whereas the protein rbST is broken down in the gut and not absorbed.

It needs to be made clear that hormones have always existed in meat. We have been ingesting these hormones without questioning the effects they might have on humans ever since mankind became meat eaters. Only recently have we become aware of hormones and their actions, and only relatively recently have steroid

53

hormones been used in agriculture. The question is whether the use of steroid hormones has any effect on the humans who consume the meat.

The three hormones, estradiol, progesterone, and testosterone, are produced naturally in cattle. Zeranol, trenbolone acetate, and melengestrol are synthetic hormones not found in cattle. The good news is that estradiol, progesterone, and testosterone are metabolized relatively quickly in the cattle, so the meat from cattle given these hormones has essentially the same amount of hormone residue as the untreated cattle meat. The hormones zeranol, melengestrol acetate, and trenbolone acetate are not metabolized as quickly, so the FDA required that manufacturers of the implantable hormones demonstrate that any residual levels in meat be well below "safe levels."

It is important to understand that the natural hormones used in cattle—estradiol, progesterone, and testosterone—are also hormones made in the human body in much higher amounts than any residuals found in meat. To put things into perspective, we need to know how much of these hormones our bodies make compared to the extra we may be getting in our meat. The average amount of estradiol found in a three ounce serving of hormone-treated meat is 1.9 nanograms as compared to 1.2 nanograms found in the meat from untreated cattle. That is an infinitesimally small difference. The amount of estradiol made in the average human female in a day is 480,000 nanograms; human males make about 136,000 nanograms a day. The effect of possibly ingesting one pound of treated meat a day, or eating an extra 3.5 nanograms of estradiol, is clearly too small to have any hormonal effect on adults. But what about the effect on children who eat treated meat? Children are much smaller and do not produce hormones anywhere near adult levels. Will the amount of hormone they ingest in meat have a negative effect on them? The average amount of estradiol a pre-pubertal girl produces is about 31,000 nanograms, and in pre-pubertal boys it is about 6000 nanograms. So even if a child were to ingest one pound of meat a day, the amount of "extra" estradiol from meat consumption would be insignificant.

We can take this evaluation of estrogen in our diet one step further and look at the other foods containing estrogens that we have been eating for centuries. We are exposed to hormones in many different foods and in varying degrees. Eggs contain 1,750 nanograms of estrogens, much more than any three ounce portion of beef. The milk from an *untreated* cow contains more estradiol than beef. We have not even talked about all the phytoestrogens that humans consume. Phytoestrogens are plant estrogens that can mimic the effects of human hormone. These plant hormones are ingested at levels 1000 fold greater than the hormones in meat. It is safe to say that humans have been consuming phytoestrogens for thousands of years without any untoward side effects. The estrogens consumed in meat are just too low, even in hormonally treated cows, to have any possible effects on humans. The same holds true for progesterone and testosterone, but estrogen tends to be the more worrisome hormone.

We have not completed the story without discussing the synthetic hormone residues (zeranol, trenbolone, and melengesterol) found in meat. These are not naturally occurring and therefore do not have a long history of being ingested by humans. Let me start by saying that melengestrol does not have data on its toxic potential, but no residual levels have been *detected* in animals. I will leave that statement alone because I have more to say about the other hormones.

According to studies on zeranol, trenbolone, and their active metabolites, lab animals developed tumors when exposed to high doses of these steroids. However, at low dose exposure they did not cause tumor growth in lab animals. As we have seen, many toxic chemicals can be benign at low doses. The high dose animal studies do not necessarily translate into human cancer, so we have to be careful when using the research information.

Eating beef that may increase our synthetic hormone exposure *possibly* leading to an increased risk of cancer is not the only problem that needs further research. Some studies have shown effects of these synthetic hormones on the developing fetus. One study showed that women who consumed beef seven or more times a week gave birth to children with lower sperm counts and possible future fertility problems. Now, of course, eating beef more than seven times a week is not advisable for anyone, even without considering the possible hormone exposure!

The FDA has studied the intake of meats treated with hormones and has found no adverse affect on humans. There have not been any studies that *conclusively* proved that hormone-treated meat has a detrimental effect on children or adults. However, medical experts tell us that there are other health reasons to limit red meat intake other than trying to avoid the miniscule possibility of hormone exposure.

My recommendation is to limit red meat intake for health reasons other than to avoid the hormone exposure. Pregnant women should especially limit intake of beef given the unknown result of zeranol or trenbolone and their metabolites on the developing fetus.

7

Are There Antibiotics in the Food We Consume and What Effects Will They Have on Us?

Antibiotics save lives, but when used incorrectly they can cause more harm than good. In contrast to hormones, antibiotic use is not restricted to cattle and sheep. Antibiotics are also used in poultry and swine, which may potentially expose many more people to unnecessary chemical exposure.

The good news is the FDA has set up strict guidelines that have to be followed when using antibiotics in animals. Tolerance levels have been set up for all antibiotics used in animals. The tolerance levels are the maximum drug concentration allowed in the animal at the time of slaughter. The tolerance levels set up by the FDA are based on potential risk to human health. For example, the antibiotic chloramphenicol used in the past was shown to cause aplastic anemia (a serious blood disorder) in humans. The exposure to the antibiotic was not dose related, so even low levels of exposure in foods could cause this fatal disease. This drug is no longer used in animals because of the potential risk to humans.

Let's take a look at the safeguards set up to protect the consumer. Farmers who raise animals for consumption must withdraw all use of any antibiotic before the animal is harvested. This is to ensure low levels of antibiotic and antibiotic metabolites in the food. The FDA regularly checks levels of antibiotic residues in foods to ensure that the guidelines for proper use of the antibiotic are being followed. They also screen for residual antibiotic levels in the slaughtered animals. Most of the time when unacceptably high levels are found in the animals, it is because of unintentional misuse of the antibiotic caused by miscommunication between agricultural workers. Accidental misuse of the antibiotic, such as not waiting the required time for withdrawal of the antibiotic before slaughter, or using too much of the antibiotic, can mean a great loss of income for the farmer if it is discovered that he has not adhered to the guidelines. This can result in government fines and the loss of the animal commodity, but the FDA guidelines must be followed to protect the health of society.

Any possible residue of antibiotics in foods can be destroyed or lessened by cooking, freezing and washing. The antibiotic levels in food are low to start with. Thus, if they are mostly destroyed from food processing and cooking, these residues do not appear to be a threat to us by causing significant drug resistance in humans. In fact, it would seem that they have virtually no effect on humans at all because we are talking about residues in the parts per million.

It appears that the possibility of eating miniscule levels of antibiotics will probably not do any harm to humans. *However,* I am much more concerned about how the antibiotics are used in the animals and the effect of that use on human health. At the present time, 70-80% of all antibiotics used are used in the animal industry. They are given to the animals in feed or water to promote growth and to decrease infection risk in the animal. Ninety percent of antibiotics used in agriculture are used to promote growth or are given to prevent infection, NOT to treat an infection. This is where the problem lies.

This non-therapeutic use of antibiotics in livestock is causing a rise in highly resistant bacteria. These "super bugs" can be and are being transmitted to humans through food and animal waste. We have seen the result of consuming foods contaminated with bacteria. Luckily, at the present time, most of these infections can be treated. However, with the sloppy use of antibiotics in the animal industry, these bacteria are becoming more resistant to treatment. This will ultimately lead to infections that cannot be treated with an antibiotic.

The overuse of antibiotics in animals causes selection of resistant bacteria. Humans can then be colonized or infected with bacteria that are resistant to the antibiotics that were used in the animals. The development of resistance to the antibiotics used in the animals could eliminate multiple classes of antibiotics used for humans that are needed to treat infections. We have seen this with resistant cases of salmonella, campylobacter, and e. coli which are dangerous gastrointestinal infections. Those are just a few of the dangerous, resistant bacteria that are emerging from inappropriate use of antibiotics in the animal industry. I am sure there will be many more resistant bacteria to emerge from the indiscriminate use of antibiotics.

Eating meat that has been treated with antibiotics does not appear to have any undue risk for the individual. This is because the FDA regulations placed on the residual antibiotic levels in the animals, along with the continued destruction of the antibiotics from heat or freezing, leaves miniscule traces of antibiotic in the meat we eat.

But unfortunately, the unrestricted use of antibiotics in the animals to prevent infection is a situation that is very dangerous! Antibiotic use in animals should be restricted to therapeutic uses. This is crucial if we are to continue to successfully treat bacterial infections in humans as well as animals. Financial gain from increasing beef or poultry production is not worth the risk of colonizing the world with super bacteria.

8

Pesticides: What Are They Good For?

Pesticides, when used judiciously, serve an excellent purpose, although they generate fear and controversy because of the toxic potential. The use of pesticides has helped to bring humans into the 21st century with less disease and more food. Pesticide usage alone has made more fresh foods available worldwide and squelched many diseases caused by vector spread. There are other advantages to pesticide usage, but I will concentrate on these main advantages.

Pesticides limit the transmission of diseases by killing insect or rodent vectors. Millions of lives have been saved because of pesticide use by limiting the spread of diseases such as malaria, plague, dengue fever, and leishmaniasis, to name just a few. Another example of the use of chemicals to maintain health is the use of chlorine, which is added to our water supply to kill bacteria that if ingested could potentially kill many people.

New diseases are popping up that could cause a pandemic of death the likes of which humans have never seen. In the past few years we have seen a number of new infectious agents develop, such as the avian flu virus, Ebola virus, west Nile virus and Hantavirus. Some of these diseases are transmitted through insects or rodents. The control of these vectors is essential to limiting the spread of disease. Pesticides are still one of the more effective means of controlling transmission of disease.

Pesticides have become essential for public health and are generally not used alone to contain infestation. Vectors of disease adapt easily when continually bombarded with the same method of control. They learn how to survive and become resistant to the method used to control them. Therefore, the use of different methods to kill an invading organism is often used. Keeping ahead of disease-spreading vectors through the use of pesticides is essential to maintaining the quality of life that we have already achieved.

Another essential advantage of the use of pesticides is the increase of the availability of foods around the world. Pesticides help to increase the yield of crops by controlling pest infestation and killing plant eating insects. By helping to decrease the loss of crops to insects and plant disease, there is an increase in the availability of fruits and vegetables throughout the world.

Infestations from plant eating insects can be kept under control by using pesticides. For example, the Mediterranean fruit fly is capable of wiping out a fruit or vegetable crop if not kept under control. Honey bees, which are essential for crop pollination, are plagued by a parasitic mite that kills the honey bee. Farmers use pesticides to kill the mite but without harming the honey bees. The honey bees are then plentiful and can continue to pollinate and produce foods.

Believe it or not, the pesticides that are used in agriculture actually save lives by allowing more food to be produced. People worldwide will be more likely to enjoy the benefits of eating plant nutrients on a regular basis. It is an obvious follow through that fewer people will die of starvation if the world is able to produce more foods to consume, but it is not so obvious to think that pesticides will decrease the risk of death from chronic diseases.

Medical studies have continually revealed that the consistent consumption of fruits and vegetables is associated with a decreased risk of heart disease, cancers, obesity, type II diabetes, and stroke. The World Health Organization (WHO) estimates that 2.7 million deaths occur each year because of low fruit and vegetable intake. A top 10 risk of global mortality is low fruit and vegetable intake! It has been estimated that 19% of gastrointestinal cancers, 31% of heart disease, and 11% of strokes are solely due to low intake of fruits and vegetables.

These studies have been consistently reproduced through research. Therefore, it seems that the use of pesticides, by increasing the food supply and plant nutrients available to the population, has the potential to lower the incidence of diseases.

There is, unfortunately, another side of pesticide use: toxic exposures. It is clear that chemical pesticides are potentially very dangerous. Toxic exposures may occur in people who work in fields that use or manufacture chemical pesticides. Some of these exposures can lead to death. Agricultural workers have an increased risk for exposure to these chemicals on a regular basis. It has been shown that because of this chronic exposure these workers have an increased rate of certain cancers and give birth to children with more birth defects and neurological and developmental problems. However, the exposure that agricultural workers encounter is much more dangerous than the average consumer. They may get the pesticide directly on their skin or inhale the pesticide on a chronic basis. These types of exposures bypass our natural detoxification mechanisms in our intestine and liver when there are large-dose exposures over a long period of time. When large doses of almost any chemical or drug occurs (even in therapeutic chemicals such as ibuprofen, a chemical used every day in children) it overwhelms our detoxification system and then can do damage to the body.

Thank goodness the body is well equipped with detoxification avenues. We have detoxification mechanisms such as anti-oxidants that are made in the body to fend off free radical damage. Toxins can be excreted from the body through liver or intestinal cells. The linings of our mouth, esophagus, stomach, skin, lung, and intestine can all be shed in the effort to destroy, neutralize or get rid of external toxin exposure. The human ability to detoxify chemicals is *not* specific, but general; in other words, we are able to detoxify many substances from many different classes of chemicals. This enables us to tackle whatever comes our way. Whether we are exposed to manmade or nature-made toxins, our bodies will do what they need to keep it from being harmed.

If we could end pesticide usage and guarantee that diseases like malaria and plague would not become rampant because of vector overgrowth, and if we could guarantee enough fruits and vegetables for the world, then doing away with pesticides in our environment would make sense. After all, we have been on this planet for millions of years and survived without the use of manmade pesticides. The problem is that we can't compare then and now. If we want to go back to the days when we took great risk by just eating food, or died of rampant vector borne diseases, or died of starvation, then it would be easy to get rid of pesticides. At the present time, however, doing away with pesticides will end up putting many more people at risk for a myriad of diseases. We need to come up with more natural ways to control pests—ones that are not going to do any harm even at higher dose exposures.

Section III

Sugar and Artificial Sweeteners

Sugar has become an evil word over the past few decades, mainly because of a gluttonous attraction to its taste. Instead of ingesting sugar in moderation, many people eat too much of it with resultant negative effects. The recommended *maximum* amount of simple sugar intake is 1–1.5 ounces per day. The average American consumes almost six times that amount in a day! Sugar has been blamed for causing food addictions, the obesity epidemic, mood disorders, arthritis, heart disease, gallstones, tooth decay, cancer, diabetes, and more. Sugar has even been called a poison. While there is a lot to be said about avoiding too much sugar, it is a misunderstood group of chemicals. People are becoming much more aware of the sugar content of foods but this "awareness" has led to more misunderstanding about sugar than true knowledge.

A relatively new set of foods are the artificial sweeteners that researchers have actively searched for or randomly stumbled upon in the laboratory. These new sweeteners carry the sweetness of sugar without the calories or resultant physiological response of sugar. Therefore, these artificial sweeteners have helped thousands of diabetics who use the "fake" version without the dangerous consequences of real sugar. Each of the artificial sweeteners have had a finger pointed at it at one time or another accusing it of causing cancer or making toxins in our bodies as a result of our metabolism of the sweetener. These artificial sweeteners are

65

appearing in all types of foods and beverages including foods eaten by babies, making the story behind artificial sweeteners an important one to know.

9

What Is Sugar?

People often think of sugar only as the substance put on cereal or in coffee to add sweetness, but there are many different types of sugar. A single sugar molecule generally refers to a molecule of glucose, fructose or galactose. When two single sugars are put together, sucrose (table sugar), lactose (milk sugar) and maltose are formed. Many single sugars together make up carbohydrates in the form of fiber and starches. You might be surprised to find out that fiber and starches are made up of single sugar molecules. There is, however, a major difference when we eat a food filled with fiber versus a food filled with simple sugars.

Simple sugars are single or double sugar molecules. They include glucose, fructose, galactose (single molecules) and maltose, sucrose, or lactose (double molecules). The amount of sugar listed on a nutrition label is the amount of *simple sugars* in the food. The simple sugars can be added in during processing or are a natural part of the food. Take a look at a carton of milk. You may be very surprised to find out that milk has 12 grams of simple sugar in an 8 ounce glass. This "sugar" is a natural milk sugar called lactose. The added sugars in the form of corn syrup, high fructose corn syrup, sucrose and honey are the sugars consumers need to notice.

People who are health conscious or need to watch their intake of simple sugars are used to looking at nutrition labels. But many people who are not used to looking at nutrition labels read the carbohydrate content of a food thinking it is the sugar content. Reading labels is an excellent idea, but it is important to understand the information on the label. The carbohydrate content includes the larger sugar molecules that make up the food, including fiber. The carbohydrate content also includes the simple sugar content and for the purpose of this chapter we are only talking about simple sugars.

How much simple sugar is too much and why is too much not a good thing? We will talk about the sugars added to foods and what to look for on labels. Sugar is put in foods in different forms, so it is important to know what to look for.

Let's start with the sugar substance that we call table sugar (sucrose). Sucrose is made mainly from the sugar cane plant and has been cultivated for thousands of years. Some table sugar is extracted from beet root as well. There is no real difference in the sugar extracted from either plant. Sucrose is extracted from the plants while leaving behind all the vitamins, minerals and fiber. It is a completely processed substance. The original state of the cane plant has no resemblance to the final product of table sugar.

Sucrose is a molecule of glucose connected to a molecule of fructose. Since sucrose is devoid of vitamins and minerals the body actually uses up vitamins and minerals to digest the sucrose and utilize it for energy.

Next we will talk about high fructose corn syrup (HFCS). There has been a lot of press on high fructose corn syrup; some authorities are even blaming it for the obesity epidemic. HFCS is a thick syrupy mixture formed from corn. There are two main types of HFCS used in processed foods. One mixture contains 55% fructose and 45% glucose or HFCS 55 that is as sweet as sucrose. Another commonly used form contains 42% fructose that is not as sweet as sucrose. The syrup is used in many foods and drinks because it is cheaper than sucrose and tends to have a longer shelf life when added to processed foods.

Next on the list is honey. Everyone thinks of honey as a natural food. It is indeed natural, but the honey we buy in the stores has been processed and clarified, so any extra benefit that the natural honey had was taken out during processing. Honey contains

31% glucose, 38% fructose with maltose, sucrose and other complex carbohydrates making up the rest of the components.

Pure maple syrup is extracted from maple trees. The syrup contains about 66% sucrose with the rest of the content being fructose, glucose, vitamins and minerals. Real maple syrup is an excellent source of manganese and zinc. Both zinc and manganese are minerals required by the body and help it fend off free radical damage. This is in contrast to the syrup that most of us purchase in the stores. It is not real maple syrup. It is instead a mixture of high fructose corn syrup and artificial maple flavoring. There are advantages to eating maple syrup, but not when eating artificial syrup.

Evaporated cane juice is another way that manufactures add sweetness to foods. Cane juice is the fluid from the cane plant that is in a less processed state than white sugar. Therefore, it retains some nutritious ingredients. Evaporated cane juice has about 66% sucrose while the rest is glucose and fructose.

In the following section we will talk about what the individual sugars do in your body so that when you read a food label you will not only understand what sugars are in the food, but how it is affecting your body. This will help those people who merely look at the label and assume all sugar is the same.

10

What Effect Does Sugar Have on the Body?

Every cell in the body needs the simple sugar, glucose, for fuel. The weak, light headed feeling that some people feel if they have skipped a meal is caused by a drop in blood glucose. The body will try to maintain a glucose level to supply the body even when we have not eaten. It will do this by metabolizing stored glucose in the liver (glycogen) and then moving on to muscle proteins and fats. The fats and proteins from muscles are broken down and used as an energy source.

Eating is a pleasurable experience for humans, but, as with most things, too much is not a good thing. Let's take a look at what happens to the sugars we eat. After a meal most of the carbohydrates that we consume get broken down to glucose; glucose is absorbed into the blood stream and causes the insulin level to go up. The more simple sugars ingested in a meal, the more rapid the rise in glucose with a greater rise in insulin. Insulin is a hormone that closely regulates glucose levels in the blood. Glucose requires this hormone to get into the cells for energy use. Insulin also stimulates glycogen storage (storage form of glucose) in the liver as well as fat production. At the same time, the body's leptin level (satiety hormone) goes up to tell the body that it is satisfied and to stop eating. The ghrelin level (hormone telling us to eat) goes down and stops giving us signals to eat. There are many more hormonal effects that the body undergoes after ingesting a meal, but we will stick to the basics of simple sugar metabolism.

The glucose that is needed for cellular metabolism is used by the body and the excess is taken up by the liver and converted to storage glucose (glycogen) to be used during times of fasting. The liver is the only organ that can make glucose when the rest of the body needs it; glucose has a two-way ticket in the liver. The excess glucose may also be converted into fat for storage and used later on.

These facts are important if we are to understand the consequences of eating too much sugar. The average individual eats 2–3 pounds of sugar per week. At the turn of the century the average sugar intake was 5 pounds per YEAR! The recommended intake of sugar should be less than 10% of calories consumed. For most of us this is between 40–55 grams of sugar per day.

Fructose is consumed in very high amounts today as compared to our ancestors. The fructose content of their diet was much lower than the average individual in the 21st century. This may be one of the reasons that humans can't handle high amounts of fructose in the diet. For example, the fructose content of an apple is about 5–7 % and fruits were the main source of fructose for our ancestors. As I stated above, many foods contain high fructose corn syrup with 55% fructose, which is a lot more than our ancestors ate. Since our genetic material has not been able to change quickly enough to adapt to this sudden increase in fructose ingestion, we are not well equipped to handle large amounts of fructose.

The body's ability to handle fructose is very different from how it handles glucose. First of all, fructose cannot be picked up by any other cell in the body except the liver (and sperm cells), whereas glucose can enter every cell in the body with the aid of insulin. This means that all the fructose we eat goes directly to the liver. The other cells in the body can't use fructose as a fuel source so it has to go the liver to be converted to a form that can somehow be utilized by the body.

Secondly, unlike glucose, fructose has a one-way ticket into the liver. Once it goes in, it can't come out. This causes the liver to rapidly metabolize the fructose. The fructose is broken down, with some of it converted to glucose, but most of it is converted into fatty acids. These fatty acids raise the serum triglyceride levels. Medical evidence has proven a link between elevated triglyceride levels and atherosclerosis, which increases risk for heart disease and stroke.

The body's hormonal response to fructose is also different from its response to glucose. The insulin level does NOT go up in response to fructose ingestion and the ghrelin and leptin levels do not change appropriately. These aberrant hormonal responses from fructose ingestion do NOT cause the proper appetite suppression from eating. This lack of appetite suppression contributes to over-eating. In other words when we eat foods with a high fructose content, they do not satisfy hunger.

Let's take a look at what happens when we drink a glass of milk. A glass of milk contains 12 grams of sugar all in the form of lactose. Lactose is made up of one glucose molecule and one galactose molecule. Unlike fructose, galactose can be taken up by many cells of the body to be utilized as fuel. This does not cause an overload of simple sugar molecules entering the liver. The galactose that makes it to the liver cells gets converted to glucose to be sent out as fuel for the other cells, or turned into glycogen for later use, or broken down and stored as fat. The major differences between eating lactose (glucose and galactose) and eating sucrose (fructose and glucose) or HFCS is that the body has a normal hormonal response to lactose, and the galactose can be used by many other cells for fuel. The ingestion of sucrose results in an abnormal hormonal response that causes an increase in calorie consumption. Since fructose can't be utilized by other cells in the body and the liver is the only organ that takes care of fructose (except sperm cells), most of the fructose ends up being converted in the liver to fatty acids.

11

Is Sugar Bad for Human Consumption?

The effects that sugar has on the body vary depending on the type of sugar. We must remember that glucose is required for every cell in the body to function. This discussion will address the ingestion of *sucrose (table sugar) and high fructose corn syrup.* The consumption of sugar has increased tremendously in the past century. With the advent of high fructose corn syrup, many of us are eating sugar when we are not aware of it. High fructose corn syrup seems to be hidden in many products that you would not suspect. We know that it is in cakes and cookies. It is also found in many breakfast cereals, "juices" that are not 100% fruit juice, dressings, yogurts, and I have even found it in breads claiming to be "heart healthy"!

There is some speculation that high fructose corn syrup has contributed to the obesity epidemic. Current statistics show that the average intake of table sugar has gone down while HFCS intake has gone up. As I stated before, HFCS contributes to an increase in serum triglycerides and can contribute to heart disease.

Let us look at some of the many problems that sugar has been accused of causing. I will look at each one individually to discuss the validity of the claim. There are some web sites that list over 100 problems associated with eating sugar. Some of these accusations are completely true and others are just plain ridiculous. Most of the claims are redundant and serve no purpose other than sensationalism. I will look at the most talked about claims and address them.

Sugar causes tooth decay. This is a true statement. Tooth decay is becoming a global problem and one of the main culprits is simple sugars. Fructose, which is the major molecule found in sucrose and HFCS, can be used by bacteria in the mouth (human cells cannot absorb fructose for energy). A result of the digestion of fructose in the bacterial cells in the mouth is the production of acid. The acid production causes a slow breakdown of the tooth enamel and eventual cavity formation.

Sugar causes diabetes. This statement is a misleading statement. Diabetes is the result of the body's inability to metabolize glucose either from insufficient amounts of insulin or the inability of the body to respond to the insulin produced. For diabetics this causes an elevated glucose level in the blood when food is ingested. People without diabetes do not have elevated glucose levels. The healthy body does not let glucose levels go up unchecked after a meal. Therefore, ingesting sugar does not cause diabetes. If it did, we could assume that the whole population would have diabetes.

Ingesting EXCESS sugar on a regular basis, however, can cause obesity. Obesity and lack of exercise are the biggest risk factors for the development of type II diabetes. Ninety percent of people with diabetes have type II. This is when the body does not respond properly to the insulin produced in the body. Type I diabetes makes up the rest of the diabetics and is caused by insufficient insulin production. As you can see, ingesting sugar is not the risk factor, although ingesting excess sugar can lead to increased weight gain and the subsequent problems associated with obesity. Some well-known complications of diabetes (not just sugar intake) are kidney disease, neuropathy (nerve damage), eye disease resulting in blindness, heart disease, strokes, and loss of limbs.

Sugar causes arthritis. This is a false statement. Sugar does not cause arthritis. Arthritis has many variables. As we age our cartilage wears down and the joints are more at risk for inflammation and arthritis. Genetics most likely plays a role in the development of arthritis, but to an unknown extent. Previous bone injuries put the joint at risk for arthritis. A myriad of autoimmune diseases also cause arthritis. Another risk factor for the development of arthritis is obesity. The chronic stress on the joints from excessive weight causes the joint to wear down. The connection with sugar is related to becoming obese. With greater sugar intake a person is more likely to become overweight, which then increases the risk of developing arthritis.

Sugar causes obesity and overweight. This is true when sugar is chronically eaten in excess and does not require further explanation.

Sugar suppresses the immune system. This statement is misleading. Excessively *high* levels of glucose that are seen in people with diabetes cause a large number of physiologic changes that predisposes them to infection. There are far too many biochemical alterations to describe here. Fortunately, most people do not walk around with excessively elevated levels of glucose. Even for those of us who do not have diabetes, just a transient elevation of glucose can have an effect on the immune system. Let me explain. Vitamin C is used by immune cells to help kill bacteria and viruses. When glucose is elevated it competes with the vitamin C that needs to enter into cells to fight off infection. This leaves the body more at risk for infection because less vitamin C is available inside the immune cell to function properly and to fight off infection. This occurs with chronically elevated levels of glucose seen in individuals with diabetes or during a transient elevation of glucose outside normal range. It is not the sugar molecule that is causing the immune dysfunction, but elevated levels outside normal range that causes a cascade of events leading to immune dysfunction.

Sugar causes heart disease. This is more true than misleading. As I have stated, the body is not well equipped to metabolize fructose. Excess fructose intake leads to an increase in serum fatty acids, which results in a higher risk for atherosclerosis (clogged arteries). If the arteries that become clogged are supplying blood to the heart, this results in heart disease. So there is an association between fructose intake and heart disease. The association of excess sugar and diabetes can also lead to heart disease.

Sugar causes headaches and migraines. This statement might be true in some people. People may have sensitivities to foods which might trigger a migraine. Individuals that suffer from migraines know exactly which foods or food additives may trigger a migraine. Sucrose or HFCS may be one of them. However, this is a very rare trigger. Hypoglycemia or low blood sugar is a more common problem for many people. Low blood sugar may result from prolonged fasting with decreased body fat stores. Low blood sugar may also occur as a result of a large simple sugar meal or snack. The body's blood glucose goes up rapidly when simple sugars make up a large part of a meal. The insulin level elevates in response to a rise in blood glucose. The rapid rise in insulin causes the blood glucose level to drop quickly. This causes the feeling of "crashing" after a sugary meal and can cause a headache.

Sugar causes hyperactivity and anxiety. This statement is addressed in a following chapter.

Sugar causes cancer. This is a false statement. All cells require glucose for energy. Cancer cells are very highly metabolic and utilize more glucose because of their excess activity. Glucose does not cause cancer; however, the cancer cells do rely on glucose for energy.

There are more sugar accusations that I could talk about but it could take up the rest of the book. I addressed the most pertinent accusations.

It seems obvious that often sugar is not good for the human body, especially when consumed in excess. However, it is important to remember that I am using the word "sugar" to represent only sucrose and HFCS. Glucose, galactose, maltose, and lactose also make up the sugar category. As I have explained, the latter do not have the same negative effects in the body as sucrose and HFCS. I recommend limiting sucrose and avoiding high fructose corn syrup intake. Excess consumption of these sugars cause many problems either directly or indirectly.

12

Does Sugar Make My Child Hyperactive?

We have all heard the terms "sugar high" and "sugar rush." They are used to refer to the physical state, which is a hyperactive or energetic state, that occurs after a person has consumed some sugary foods. Many people believe that ingesting sugar makes individuals more active. A more common idea that many parents have is that sugar affects their child's behavior making them more aggressive, or more active, or lessens their ability to concentrate.

The concept that food affects behavior is not a new idea. It has been around since the beginning of the century. The '70s brought us the Feingold diet; this is a diet that restricted food additives, food colorings, and sugar in an effort to treat behavioral disorders. This diet has been studied and has never been proven to be effective, but the idea that limiting sugar intake to help behavior has perpetuated. The misinformation chain is at play here. The idea that hyperactivity and sugar are intimately connected has not fallen out of favor despite evidence to prove otherwise.

There are some issues that need to be teased out before we can comment on whether sugar affects activity level. Studies done on children to prove or disprove the sugar hyperactivity connection are only valid if the amount of sugar given to the study subjects is specific, a control group is present, and all participants and researchers are unaware of which child received sugar or placebo. This is called a double-blind placebo-controlled study. There have been many studies that meet these criteria of validity and these studies have proved that when children are given sucrose they *do not become more active.*

The perception that sugar causes hyperactivity still persists despite science proving it wrong. Could it be the parent's expectation that their child becomes hyper after sugar ingestion? Do parents who are less able to cope with a child being normally active and playful have a need to blame it on something?

A study looking at parents' perceptions of children's activity after "sugar" ingestion was undertaken. In this study the children were all given a sugar substitute without the parents being aware of this information. The parents, who were told their children received sucrose, reported worsening behavior and increased activity even though their children were not given sucrose. This tells us that it was the parents who perceived that their children were displaying increased activity rather than a true increase in activity. A possibility for this misperception may be because of the circumstances during which children tend to eat sugary foods. This includes parties and play dates. Children are naturally more active when they are with other children and although sweet junk foods may be ingested, sugar has nothing to do with their increased level of activity.

When we understand the effects of sugar on the brain it will lead us to a better expectation of what happens to us when we eat. Let us take a look at the effects of glucose and fructose on the brain. Remember these are the simple sugars that come together to make sucrose.

Since fructose does not cross the blood-brain barrier, nor does it raise the insulin level, it would appear that it does not play a significant role in the story of sugar and hyperactivity. However, because fructose is converted to glucose, it does have an indirect effect on the brain by way of glucose. Let's take a closer look at the effect of glucose. Glucose, as well as insulin, crosses the blood brain barrier and therefore may have dramatic effects on the brain.

The proof that sugar does not cause increased activity is in the science of the brain. Glucose causes an inhibitory effect on certain glucose-sensitive brain cells. These cells secrete proteins called orexins when they are stimulated. Orexins are protein molecules in the brain that stimulate wakefulness and energy expenditure. When the body has a meal, the serum glucose rises and the brain decreases the production of orexins, which makes the body more tired! We all know this feeling of being tired after eating a meal and this is the reason why. When the glucose level drops slightly during fasting, the orexin level rises and makes the body more awake in an effort to get food.

This all makes perfect sense. The fluctuations in blood glucose levels do affect activity, but not the way most people have thought for all these years. The chemistry of the brain shows us the truth. The body is continually trying to survive. When food is scarce and the blood sugar goes lower, the brain activates us to search for food so we do not starve. These minor fluctuations in blood sugar have major effects on our brain, all in an effort to keep us alive.

There certainly are people who are more sensitive than others to fasting and sugar intake. Some people can go hours without eating and suffer no ill effects. They can work right through lunch and never feel weak, light headed, tired, and/or dizzy because of a dip in blood sugar. Their body is well equipped to maintain the blood glucose level. Then there are some people, who, if forced to skip lunch because of time constraints, feel the slight dip in blood sugar (the body tries to maintain the glucose level at all costs) and manifest a host of unpleasant symptoms such as weakness, tremulousness, dizziness, or even feelings of faintness. Children tend to react differently from adults to many situations, and dips in blood sugar are no exception. Whereas some adults may get weak from a slight dip in serum glucose, some children can become hyperactive, cranky, and aggressive.

You may be thinking: how does this explain the perception of increased activity from a sugary meal? Children (and adults for that matter) who ingest a high sugar meal may have significant dips in serum glucose because of an excessive swing in insulin. The sugar load from a high simple sugar meal causes a quick spike in serum insulin with a subsequent rapid decline in glucose. This dip in blood sugar and the accompanying behavior changes may result in the perception that sugar is making a child hyper. Instead, what is happening is that the body is responding to the low blood sugar causing some children to become aggressive and hyperactive instead of weak.

There are people who may swear that sugar makes their children more active. They may even feel that sugar makes *them* more active. There is a good explanation for adults or even children feeling more active after a meal. There are children and adults who do not do well with prolonged periods between meals because of a dropping blood sugar. When this occurs a weak feeling occurs and the body craves food. The desire to eat foods that will rapidly increase the glucose level is very strong. Once food is ingested, the weak feeling will disappear and energy levels will be restored. The low glucose feeling is a very unpleasant feeling, while the restoring of normal glucose levels is a wonderful feeling. As the weak feeling dissipates, our energy levels slowly come back to normal. This may be perceived as a "sugar rush," when it is really just a slightly aberrant response to glucose fluctuations.

13

Is Sugar Addicting?

Eating food is a very pleasurable experience. For many people, eating sweet foods is even more pleasurable. The feeling of needing to eat something sweet is not an unusual one. Many of us feel incomplete after a meal if it is not followed by a sweet-tasting food or drink. Why does this occur? Are humans addicted to sweetness and sugar? Most authorities feel that sugar is not physically addicting but is merely psychologically addicting. They argue that the urge to eat sweets is a learned behavior, and people who consume sugar in excess have developed this bad habit over time. In recent years studies have been coming out that challenge this thought process.

Many people who are reading this book know all too well the craving for something sweet. This feels very much like a physical reaction, not a learned desire. The nagging sensation or incomplete feeling is very real and does not disappear until something sweet is ingested. Recent research is delving into sugar and its effect on the human body, in particular the effect on the brain.

Before the invention of supermarkets and processed foods, our ancestors had to go out to collect foods from the environment. They had to learn which foods were safe to eat and which were potentially dangerous. The sweet taste of foods generally meant that the food was safe to eat. A bitter or biting taste usually meant more danger and the likelihood that the food would be harmful if ingested. So the urge to eat sweet food is probably a survival mechanism encoded somewhere in our DNA. We don't need these "sweet genes" to survive in today's world, but too short a time has gone by for the genes to disappear. This leaves us with the survival mechanism to eat sweets in this sweet-laden society.

There is interesting new data about glucose and its effect on the brain. Experiments with rats have identified withdrawal symptoms after given a high glucose diet. When the sugar was withdrawn from the diet, the rats experienced behavioral changes and decreased body temperature, similar to symptoms of withdrawal from opioids (such as heroine and morphine). Sugar-dependant rats have brain changes similar to a morphine addicted brain, and it has since been shown that the characteristics of a brain craving sugar are similar to a drug-addicted brain.

Ingestion of sucrose releases endogenous opioids while insulin blocks the release of the feel-good hormones. Many of us can attest to that pleasing satisfaction after eating a dessert. To further prove the association of sucrose and opioid stimulation, a study was done on bulimic girls. Bulimics will binge on high sugar and high fat foods. The study involved giving the girls an opioid blocking drug. When the girls were on the drug, their sweet binging was decreased by 50%. Other studies have shown that when research animals are given opioid receptor-blocking medication, they were significantly less interested in eating.

Does this research mean that we are addicted to sugar or that we just feel good when we consume it? The research seems to be pointing in the direction of a possible physical mechanism that can explain a true addiction. An addiction is defined as behavioral and brain changes from increased intake as well as changes in brain chemistry and behavior from the withdrawal of the substance. More research needs to be done in this area, but all fingers seem to be pointing to sugar addiction as a real phenomenon.

14

Are Artificial Sweeteners Safe for Me and My Child?

The use of artificial sweeteners has become very popular over the last few decades. The need for humans to satisfy a sweet tooth without calories has created a need for non- caloric sweeteners. Technology has brought us many things, but who would have thought that we would be consuming massive amounts of fake sugar? The current sweeteners on the market are aspartame, sucralose, neotame, acesulfame potassium, and saccharin.

Parents often ask me if it is okay to give their child foods that contain artificial sweeteners. I always give the same answer. Children should be eating healthy fresh foods, not low calorie man-made "diet" foods. I do not want children eating foods with artificial sweeteners, but if they happen to accidently eat a food containing one of the above sweeteners, no harm will be done. Now, when I say this to an audience full of parents, I usually hear lots of rumbling and repeated questioning to make sure they heard me correctly. Some people may insist that these artificial sweeteners are causing cancer. I have to admit that the mere mention of the word saccharin still sends chills up and down my spine. I grew up in the '70s when all the "controversy" surrounding saccharin and cancer was at a peak. I have been part of the misinformation chain. The idea that saccharin causes cancer was so big that it became part of the pop culture of my adolescent years. On the following pages I will evaluate each of the commonly used sweeteners and possibly dispel common beliefs perpetuated in the misinformation chain.

Aspartame was discovered accidentally in 1963. It was found to be 200 times sweeter than sugar. Aspartame is made from two amino acids (protein building blocks), phenylalanine and aspartic acid. When it is metabolized in the body it gets broken down to the original amino acids and methanol. There has been a lot of "noise" surrounding the use of aspartame. Many people lodged complaints about possible allergic reactions, headaches or neurological reactions. Studies started to come out shortly after aspartame was FDA approved, blaming it on an increased rate of brain tumors. Even the FDA approval of aspartame was controversial; some people have said that it was approved as a political favor and was not approved based on good science.

The possibility that some people are more sensitive to aspartame does exist. People who have had adverse reactions to this sweetener should avoid it. That is simple enough. Some people react differently to different foods based on many different factors. We all know people who can't eat certain foods because of adverse reactions. They know to stay clear of the food.

The breakdown products of aspartame seems to concern some people. Two of the breakdown products, phenylalanine and aspartic acid, are both amino acids. One of the concerns about aspartame is the worry that when it becomes metabolized, it will increase serum levels of the brain chemicals serotonin, dopamine, or norepinephrine. Studies on human volunteers using low, medium, and high doses of aspartame did not show any neurologic effects from large doses of aspartame given at one time. There was no stimulatory or sedating effect from the aspartame. Eating a high protein meal contains a higher amount of phenylalanine than one or two packets of aspartame, so why are people trying to make the claim that this is a cause for concern in healthy people? I am excluding people with rare disorders of phenylalanine metabolism. Many studies have also failed to show any evidence to link aspartame to headaches or neurologic abnormalities.

The breakdown product methanol also causes concern. I have seen many web sites that are very emphatic about touting the dangers of aspartame and its byproduct, methanol. These types of web sites are responsible for spreading fear and misinformation.

The originators of these sites fail to ask questions or to do a proper amount of research, all in the name of sensationalism.

Methanol, also known as wood alcohol, is indeed formed by aspartame metabolism and is used in many chemical solutions. It can kill a person if taken in a large quantity. Methanol is formed when aspartame is metabolized, but only about 4 mg of methanol is produced from one packet of aspartame. What we need to realize is that methanol is made in our bodies every day; in the amount of about 300-600 mg. The metabolism of pectin found in fruits raise serum methanol levels considerably more than drinking a cup of coffee with a packet of aspartame. If our body produces methanol from normal metabolism of foods at much greater rates than from aspartame ingestion, it is a natural observation that we are well equipped to break down *small* amounts of methanol without dangerous effects.

The next controversy surrounding aspartame is the possible link to its use and brain tumors. In the 1990s it was a bit scary when it was first suggested that the incidence of brain cancer in the general population started to increase coincidently with the rise of aspartame usage. The speculation was that the aspartame was causing this increase. The accusation that aspartame was causing the increase in brain cancer was unfounded. The incidence of brain tumors in the general population was found to have increased eight years *before* aspartame was approved for use. Since then studies with rats have not shown any signs of an increased risk of brain tumors, even when using massive doses of the sweetener. However, we still don't know why the incidence of brain tumors increased in humans.

A study done in 2006 in rats showed an increased rate of leukemia and lymphomas when given aspartame at high doses. This has generated renewed controversy over the long term use of this sweetener. There are recommendations to study high dose use over a long period. When and if these studies do come out, it is crucial to remember that "the dose makes the poison." Claims may be made stating that aspartame causes cancer in lab animals. It is EXTREMELY important to look at three main areas when looking at rodent studies to answer future questions about aspartame safety. The amount of aspartame, the metabolic byproducts and the enzymes needed to make the byproducts, must be evaluated before any statement can be made in future studies. Having this information in the study will make the difference between a well-done study versus another poorly constructed study to fuel the misinformation chain.

The latest word on aspartame was a large scale review of aspartame published in the September 2007 issue of *Critical Reviews in Toxicology*. This study reviewed over 500 studies done on aspartame and concluded that there is no association with aspartame use and cancer, neurologic abnormalities, or other health problems. It has been deemed safe for human consumption!

Neotame is another sweetener that is a derivative of aspartame. Neotame was FDA approved for use in July, 2002. It is made by adding 3-dimethylbutyl to phenylalanine and aspartic acid. It is heat stable, which makes it better for cooking and is 7000-13000 times sweeter than sugar! Neotame is rapidly metabolized in the body to methanol and de-esterified neotame. There is very little research on this sweeter and lots of data on 3-dimethylbutyl, which is a hazardous chemical. I can't comment on the safety of neotame until further research is completed.

The next sweetener we will talk about is acesulfame potassium. This sweetener is 100-200 times sweeter than table sugar. It does have a slight aftertaste so it is often combined with other artificial sweeteners. It was approved for use in 1998 and is now used in over 4000 products. Acesulfame is absorbed and excreted intact. That means that there is not a significant breakdown of the chemical in the body. Ninety-nine percent of the chemical is excreted in the urine and 1% is excreted in feces. The ability of this chemical to be 100% excreted in its original form seems to be a tremendous advantage since the chemical breakdown products of other artificial sweeteners are usually the cause for concern. Any concern you may have about potassium ingestion from this sweetener should be quelled easily. A packet of acesulfame potassium contains only 10 mg of potassium, while most people need to eat about 2500 mg of potassium each day.

There have been over 90 studies looking at the possible effects of the consumption of acesulfame. To date the studies did not show any link to cancer or mutagenesis. Since there has been some criticism of these **studies** citing some possible flaws, the story does not seem to be completely finished; as always, studies will continue to attempt to refute or confirm an accusation. For now acesulfame seems safe.

Sucralose is next on our list to talk about. Sucralose is commonly known as Splenda®. It is formed by replacing three molecules on table sugar (sucrose) with chlorine molecules. It is 600 times sweeter than sugar and very stable at various temperatures. This allows it to be useful for cooking. It was approved by the FDA in 1998 and is currently found in thousands of foods.

Sucralose is not absorbed fully after oral intake. The body does not recognize sucralose as a sugar and therefore it has none of the metabolic consequences of eating sugar. Most of the compound is excreted unchanged through the gastrointestinal tract. According to human studies about 15% of it is absorbed; of this 15% about 40% is metabolized and broken down. That means that roughly 6% of sucralose is metabolized after ingestion. Everything else is excreted unchanged.

People are wary of sucralose because of the chlorine molecules. Chlorine can be found in hundreds of foods. It is usually bound to something else such as sodium that helps to keep the molecule stable and harmless. However, when chlorine and organic compounds (organochlorines) are mixed, it is a different story. The combination of chlorine and organic compounds are usually very toxic. To find out that the breakdown products of sucralose are organochlorines is not very reassuring!

The breakdown products are given the names 1, 6 DCF and 4 CG. Thank goodness there is more to this story. It turns out that not only very small amounts of 1, 6 DCF and 4 CG produced, but they are not at all toxic. This was confirmed by lab studies on monkeys. The scientists used sucralose, 1, 6 DCF, 4 CG and another organochlorine known to cause neurologic degeneration, 6 CG. They gave these chemicals to the monkeys in high doses. The 6 CG was the only substance found to cause brain lesions in the monkeys. The monkeys given sucralose and its breakdown products did not have any neurologic effects, even from high doses of these chemicals. This has helped confirm that sucralose and its metabolites are safe.

The FDA approved the use of sucralose after reviewing more than 100 studies. The studies were done to evaluate the carcinogenic potential as well as possible reproductive, neurologic, or genetic toxicities. No study has shown that there are any problems with high doses of sucralose.

It is time to talk about the oldest sweetener on the market, saccharin. It was discovered in 1878 and is 300 times sweeter than sugar but has a slightly bitter aftertaste. Saccharin does not undergo any metabolism in humans—it goes out the way it came in.

This chemical has been under investigation since 1907. The use of saccharin has waxed and waned over the past century, mainly in response to sugar shortages during the wars. Starting in the 1960s the use of saccharin increased because of the concern over diet and weight. Studies started to come out around this time about the possible link between saccharin and cancer. In 1977 a study came out linking high dose saccharin to bladder cancer in rats. The government then wanted to ban the use of saccharin, but because it was the only available non-calorie sweetener, the public pressure to keep it on the market was too great. Instead, the government mandated that a label be placed on all items containing saccharin warning that it may be carcinogenic. The immense numbers of studies that have been carried out since the label mandate have refuted any link with cancer and saccharin.

The conclusions from studies that were done on the rats in the '70s should never have been carried over to human health because the mechanism that caused the saccharin to be harmful to the rats does not exist in humans. The enzyme that converts saccharin to a dangerous compound in the rats is not present in humans, therefore making the data completely invalid! Because saccharin enters and exits our body without being metabolized, there are no other chemical byproducts that need to be evaluated.

Since then there have been numerous studies on saccharin, none of them linking saccharin to cancer. In 2000 manufacturers of food containing saccharin were not required to have any cancer warning on the label. As a matter of fact, we can say that saccharin has the longest track record of safety.

Unfortunately or fortunately, depending how you look at the situation, the negative press that saccharin has received has been ingrained in many people. I personally have never used saccharin nor have my children ever had saccharin. This is not due to any scientific conclusion that I have come to, but is merely the result of being influenced by a very misguided misinformation chain. Growing up in a time where the saccharin packets had cautions about causing cancer in lab animals has been embedded in my psyche. It just goes to show us how strong emotions can guide us, even in the face of opposing scientific data.

These sweeteners are hidden in thousands of foods. The sweeteners can be found in foods often given to babies such as yogurts and cereals. This is a reminder to all parents to read labels and to be aware of what you are feeding your children. As I said in the beginning of the chapter, children should not be eating artificial sweeteners on a regular basis.

Artificial sweeteners available for consumption are safe (for now). However they do not offer any nutritional benefits and should not be given on a regular basis to children.

Section IV

Boosting Immunity to Prevent Illness and Possibly Delaying Alzheimer's

Alzheimer's disease is not a given as we get older. It is a horrible disease where the affected individuals suffer, and everyone around them also suffers a great deal. There are families that have a greater predisposition to developing Alzheimer's, where dementia is a large part of getting older, and then there are families who have 90-year-old grandparents living alone and doing crossword puzzles to keep themselves busy. Of course genes have a lot to do with this phenomenon, but how we chose to live our lives may have an impact on the possibility of developing Alzheimer's.

The same kind of differences apply to how people react to infections. Some people are genetically more prone to getting sick than other people. The many people who are more prone to illness may often look to herbal remedies that claim to build up the immune system or, better yet, to cure the common cold—a feat scientists have been trying to accomplish since there have been scientists. There are many ways we can tank up our immune system without "turning to the strange," and the following chapters will tell how.

15

Can I Decrease My Risk of Developing Alzheimer's Disease?

How many times have you walked into a room to get something and have completely forgotten what brought you into the room? You look around the room to look for clues to jog your memory, and suddenly you remember what brought you there. This is a normal part of life for many of us, and these little acts of forgetfulness do not usually go much further.

This is not the case for five million Americans who are suffering from Alzheimer's disease (AD). The scenario usually goes like this. A person may start to forget minor things like phone numbers or addresses. As time goes on, there may be trouble remembering that last week they had a lunch date with a friend. The simplest tasks, like making a sandwich or getting dressed, start to become too difficult to accomplish. Instead of walking into a room and forgetting why they walked into the room, they start to forget where they are or even who they are. Eventually, they may no longer recognize loved ones and become completely dependent on the help of others. Many people afflicted with Alzheimer's disease may progress to this point, but is it possible to prevent this progression or even decrease the risk of acquiring this devastating disease?

Alzheimer's disease was first described by Alois Alzheimer in 1907. He described the brain pathology in two patients with the disease by examining their brains after death. He noted abnormal areas that are now called neuritic plaques and neurofibrillary tangles. Today, the diagnosis of Alzheimer's can be made confidently on the basis of clinical symptoms, although definitive diagnosis can only be made upon examination of the brain after death. The DSM IV states that the diagnosis of AD must include a gradual loss of memory along with impairment of one or more areas of cognitive function that cannot be explained by any other neurologic disease. The other cognitive problems can include apraxia, agnosia and aphasia. Apraxia is another term used for the inability to manipulate tools. When apraxia afflicts a person with AD, the ability to manipulate the environment to accomplish a task is disturbed, and daily tasks like getting toothpaste out of the tube and onto a toothbrush becomes too complicated. Agnosia is the inability to recognize people or common objects. This can present as not being able to visually recognize a toaster, microwave oven, or a deck of cards. Aphasia is the inability to use language effectively; it is the loss of understanding the meaning of words or the loss of the ability to use words to communicate thoughts. A loved one may want to eat dinner but cannot put the words together to ask to eat, or may not understand a command like "pass the salt, please." A loss of executive function may also be a part of this devastating disease. This means that planning simple tasks becomes difficult and using numbers may be impossible.

In the 1990s, the people of the United States watched as a previous leader of the free world, President Ronald Reagan, deteriorated from Alzheimer's disease. He made his disease public in 1994, when he released a hand written note in his own recognizable hand writing telling the country of his disease. At the time of his announcement, he was aware of his illness. As time went on Nancy Reagan told the world that he was unable to recognize anyone, eventually not even her. President Reagan helped to raise awareness of the disease by his courageous announcement. He also helped to lift the stigma of the disease. If someone like Ronald Reagan, who represented such strength, energy and success, could be diagnosed with Alzheimer's, it meant anyone could get the disease. The nation felt the suffering of his wife and family. Watching a loved one deteriorate mentally is heart breaking. Fortunately, with new research and therapies for Alzheimer's disease, it is very likely that fewer people in the future will suffer this fate.

We have come a long way in understanding the pathology behind this disease. Before we can go into a discussion about any possible ways to decrease risk for the disease, we need to know what causes the disease.

The proposed pathologic cascade of Alzheimer's events should be explained so that the reader can understand how the preventative measures I talk about in the following paragraphs impact on the disease.

Amyloid precursor protein (APP) is a protein manufactured in many cells in the body especially in brain cells. The protein is mainly involved in the formation of the brain cells and helps in orchestrating the communication abilities between nerve cells throughout the body. The protein is broken down by three different enzymes into different smaller protein particles. Of the three enzymes that cleave APP, two of them form a neurotoxic breakdown product called β amyloid protein and one of them forms a more harmless breakdown product. Our genetics plays a role in the activity of these enzymes, and people who have more activity in the enzymes that produce the toxic β amyloid protein are at higher risk for developing AD.

Some patients with Alzheimer's disease have a mutated form of APP rendering it more susceptible to excessive breakdown by the enzymes that produce β amyloid. β amyloid protein is insoluble, highly neurotoxic, and aggregates (clumps together) in the brain. If the APP is normal in structure, it is mainly broken down to a soluble protein that does not cause a problem.

The β amyloid protein accumulates in the brain and blood vessels of the brain. The accumulation of the protein causes inflammation around the brain cells as well as in the blood vessels. Depending on an individual's genetic propensity towards inflammation, the severity of the inflammatory reaction will vary. People more prone to inflammation reactions will have increased damage, whereas people who are genetically less inclined to have large inflammatory reactions will have less damage. Inflammation in blood vessels can lead to decreased blood flow to the vital brain tissue compounding the pathology of these patients.

The inflammatory reaction causes the formation of hydrogen peroxide, free radicals, and other mediators of cell damage. The free radical is a highly charged molecule looking for any way it can to become more stable. It does this by rapidly moving through the body and banging into cell membranes. When this occurs in the brain, along with the other mediators of inflammation, the cell membranes are damaged. There is a loss of brain cells as well as the loss of the cells' ability to communicate with one another. The pathologic end result is the formation of the neuritic plaques and neurofibrillary tangles in the brain that are the definitive diagnostic pathologic findings. The clinical end result is the slow mental deterioration of individuals until they can no longer care for themselves.

Thirty million people worldwide are afflicted with Alzheimer's disease (AD) and as the population ages this number will increase because the risk of Alzheimer's disease increases as we get older.

Alzheimer's disease can be in the form of early-onset disease that presents before age 60 and late-onset disease that presents later in life. The early-onset disease is genetically transmitted as an autosomal dominant trait. It causes 6–7% of Alzheimer's cases and unfortunately is not as modifiable as late-onset disease risk factors. Late-onset disease has one known susceptibility gene found on the apolipoprotien E gene (apo E). People who carry the apo E4 allele of this protein are at greater risk for the development of the disease. (To explain what an allele is, think of the gene for eye color; some of us have light blue eye alleles in the eye color gene, while others have all dark colors in the gene for eye color.)

Three mutations have been identified and are associated with 90% of the early onset disease that occurs before age 60. The first of the genetic transmitted AD mutations is found on chromosome 21; the gene makes the amyloid precursor protein (APP). The mutated APP, as I said above, gets cleaved excessively by the enzymes that produce the toxic β Amyloid protein. Interestingly, children with Down's syndrome have three copies of chromosome 21 (trisomy 21) and every person with Down's who lives longer than the age of 40 has the same neurologic findings as people with Alzheimer's disease. A new theory as to the etiology of later-onset Alzheimer's is the accumulation of cells in the body that contain three copies of chromosome 21. The theory supposes that there is some alteration in cell reproduction causing an increase in cells that have multiple copies of chromosomes, specifically the 21st chromosome. It has been shown that people diagnosed with Alzheimer's have a 3 to 5-fold increase in the number of trisomy 21 cells in their body, and mothers of Down's syndrome children have an increased risk for Alzheimer's. This finding may bring about a new way to help with the diagnosis of AD, checking buccal (cheek) smears for the number of trisomy 21 cells.

The other two mutations are in the genes that make presenilin proteins. The gene for presenilin 1 is found on chromosome 14 and the gene for presenilin 2 is found on chromosome 1. The presenilin proteins are involved with one of the enzymes that break down APP into β amyloid protein. The mutated presenilin gene probably causes an increased activity in the enzyme that results in more production of β amyloid which results in Alzheimer's disease. The genetic transmission of Alzheimer's disease is not a modifiable risk factor, although there are many new areas of research delving into the pathways that can be targeted for therapy.

People who carry the apo E4 allele have a 29-fold greater risk of Alzheimer's if they eat a diet high in fat (>40%) compared to people who eat a high fat diet without the apo E4 allele. It makes good sense to stick with a diet that is less than 40% fat for all of us.

There are a few non-genetic risk factors that we will talk about. The strength of association for each of the mentioned factors varies, but if all of the advice below is taken seriously, there is a potential to reduce your risk for late-onset Alzheimer's (assuming you are not genetically prone to the disease).

The number one risk factor is age. The second strongest risk factor is having a first degree relative with Alzheimer's.

People who have first degree relatives with AD have a 3 to 4-fold increase in risk of developing the disease. We can't change our family so this risk factor is non-modifiable. Getting older would at first seem to be a non-modifiable risk factor, but merely aging may not be the risk factor. The numbers show that the older we get, the more likely we are to develop dementia. The risk of Alzheimer's doubles every five years after the age of 65. Although we want to live to a ripe old age, we all want to be able to *enjoy* old age—not just arrive there. There seems to be some things we can do in our lives to help achieve that goal.

High blood pressure, also known as hypertension, increases the risk for the development of AD. Men with midlife high blood pressure were five times more likely to develop AD. The physiology behind high blood pressure and AD is mostly from inflammation. The increase arterial pressure impairs blood flow that initiates inflammation and decreases delivery of vital elements to the cells. The end result is cell damage and death. When this occurs in the brain, the cascade of events for AD ensue. One of the largest risk factors for high blood pressure is obesity. It is a natural follow through to say that maintaining a healthy weight will decrease risk for high blood pressure and AD. It also appears that obesity alone is a risk factor. This is most likely due to inflammatory damage; it is well known that obese people are loaded with inflammatory mediators as a result of an excess in fat cells. Adipose tissue (fat cells) is a hormonally active tissue and the fat cells release mediators that promote inflammation. For the many people who have essential hypertension (high blood pressure without an obvious cause) pharmacologic intervention may be necessary to keep pressure within normal range. Maintaining a blood pressure within a healthy range and decreasing risk factors that promote high blood pressure will ultimately decrease the risk for development of AD.

A very interesting association with the risk of developing AD is education level. There is a higher incidence of dementia in people without education compared to ones with a high school diploma. There are many theories as to why this association exists, but none of them are proven. One possibility is occupational exposure. Less educated individuals are more likely to be employed in jobs where exposure to pesticides and industrial toxins are increased. Other theories includes lack of brain stimulating activities, decreased social stimulation, and increased depression rates, which are all higher in less educated people.

Vascular disease has a close association with risk of Alzheimer's. Vascular disease can be caused by genetics, increased homocysteine levels, hypertension, tobacco smoking, hypercholesterolemia, and diabetes. Type II diabetes is a modifiable risk factor. Maintaining a healthy weight, regular exercise, and good eating habits, can all decrease the risk for type II diabetes development. Type I diabetes risk factor is not yet a modifiable risk factor. The elevation of the amino acid homocysteine is a known risk factor for the development of cardiovascular disease. Genetics has a hand in homocysteine levels, but making sure that vitamin B6, vitamin B12 and folate levels are maintained can decrease elevated levels. This will therefore decrease risk of cardiovascular disease, which will help decrease the risk of AD. Maintaining a good cholesterol level by eating well, exercising, and using medications when indicated is another way to reduce vascular disease risk—as well as not smoking, which does not need to be elaborated. Many of the preventative actions for vascular disease overlap and can be enhanced simply by a healthy lifestyle of eating fruits, vegetables, high fiber and performing regular exercise.

Eating a diet low in omega 3 fatty acids along with a high fat diet has a positive association with risk of Alzheimer's. I recommend eating fish high in omega 3 fatty acids for the overall health benefit with the added benefit of a reduced risk of AD.

I wish I enjoyed drinking a glass of wine each night because the beneficial effects of red wine just keep on coming. It appears that drinking one to two glasses of wine each day reduces the risk of Alzheimer's. If you drink more or less than one to two glasses a day, it voids the reduced risk of getting the disease. The most obvious reason for this effect is that the one to two glasses of wine deliver an optimal amount of disease-fighting polyphenols without the negative effects of too much alcohol. If too much alcohol is consumed, even the plentiful antioxidants cannot reverse the damaging effects of alcohol. So drink in moderation!

One of my favorite studies done on Alzheimer's disease patients looked at exercise and deterioration of mental state. I am an avid exerciser, and I try to look for all the possible benefits of exercise because, as many of you know, it can sometimes be difficult, if not painful, to keep up with a good regimen. The more positive the effects of exercise are, the easier it can be to overcome barriers to exercising. Knowing that another benefit to exercise may be decreasing Alzheimer's disease risk may help knock down a barrier to regular exercise for all of us. The study found that an exercise routine done two times a week for people already diagnosed with the disease had a significant drop in the rate of decline in mental function. A sedentary lifestyle with lack of daily activity will increase risk for AD for people not diagnosed with Alzheimer's. The benefits of physical activity are plenty and everyone should be exercising on a regular basis. Every time you go to a physician's office an inquiry should be made into how you exercise and how often. It does not matter if the patient is 3 years or 83 years old; we all have to be exercising regularly.

Another strong association with increased risk of Alzheimer's is a history of multiple incidences of head trauma, in particular a history of three or more concussions increases risk significantly. Football players are at higher risk because of multiple impacts to the head. Any type of significant head injury may set off an inflammatory reaction inside the brain. The inflammatory reaction, along with a genetic configuration that promotes inflammation, can take decades to slowly cause neuron destruction, increased plaque formation, and eventually cause AD.

The Kame Project is an excellent study that looked at fruit and vegetable juice consumption among people 65 years and older. The study participants were followed from 1994 to 2001 and were dementia free at the outset of the study. They found that participants who drank fruit or vegetable juices three or more times a week had a decreased rate of onset of AD. The benefits of drinking juices were enhanced even more with people who had risk factors like the ApoE4 allele carriers. This study did not show strength of association from vitamin C, beta-carotene, vitamin E or tea drinking.

The polyphenols in the juices act as anti-oxidants and are able to cross the blood brain barrier to protect against oxidant damage—in particular the flavonols like quercetin and kaempferol. These flavonols are found in abundance in wine, leeks, blueberries, onions, apples, and broccoli. The juices with the highest flavonol content include purple grape, cranberry, apple, and grapefruit juice. For those of you who suddenly want to start drinking grapefruit juice and are taking medications, check with your doctor first because there are compounds in this juice that may interact with certain medications.

There is one last topic I must talk about before finishing this subject, and that is the proposed association between hydrogen peroxide (H_2O_2), β-amyloid protein and Alzheimer's disease. The enzyme superoxide dismutase is the one that produces H_2O_2 from oxygen free radicals. Interestingly, the gene for this enzyme is found on chromosome 21! If you remember the theory that I mentioned before about late onset Alzheimer's disease possibly being related to the accumulation of cells with three copies of chromosome 21, the pieces of a gigantic puzzle may start to be coming together. The extra copy of chromosome 21 produces more of the enzyme superoxide dismutase compared to cells with the normal two copies of the chromosome. The extra production of superoxide dismutase causes an increase in hydrogen peroxide production with an imbalance in the oxidant/anti-oxidant ratio. This may explain why adults with Down syndrome who live past 40 years develop AD as they age. It makes sense that the more pro-oxidants there are in our brain, the more likely will be the development of inflammation with cellular damage. The more we understand about the disease, the more likely we are to find a cure.

So to sum it all up: exercise, keep mentally active, don't smoke, maintain a healthy weight, treat high blood pressure, avoid head trauma producing sports, eat an abundance of fruits and vegetables (especially the ones with a high flavonol content), drink one to two glasses of red wine daily, eat fatty fish on a regular basis and drink grape juice, apple juice, cranberry juice, or grapefruit juice at least three times a week.

16

Do Herbal Remedies Really Help to Prevent Colds and Flu?

I am going to focus only on the topic of herbal mixtures that make claims to prevent colds and flu. There is data on many different herbs for many ailments, but we are going to stick only to the colds and flu topic. Before I go on to answer the question, it is important to know what constitutes herbal supplements. They are considered dietary supplements and are not regulated by the FDA. Herbal supplements can come in extract form, pills, or teas. The herbal supplements come from plants grown in soil around the world. Since manufacturers are not required to check for contaminants in the product, a risk of ingesting environmental contaminants is introduced. This possibility was researched in a study that looked at 27 common botanicals; the researchers found 47 different contaminant metals in the products, including iron, titanium, mercury, lead, and barium!

Many herbal supplements make unsubstantiated claims of preventing illnesses citing only "one" study to attempt to back up their claim. This study is usually done by the manufacturer of the supplement.

The herbal supplements are mixtures of dry or liquid extracts from plants and weeds. Yes, there are weeds in some of these supplements that even our starving ancestors would not indulge in. Yet we flock to the stores to buy these "miracle pills" filled with dehydrated plants. It is interesting that so many people trust the manufacture of these pills. They will ingest the dried up weeds and flowers and whatever else in the hope of fighting off a cold, allevi-ating menopause or PMS symptoms, improving memory, increas-ing energy, or improving depressive symptoms. People think if the package says "all natural" it must be good. They are moving to these "natural remedies" hoping to avoid pharmaceuticals, but what many people do not realize is that these herbal remedies can cause dangerous drug interactions, allergic reactions, toxic inges-tion of metals, liver inflammation, rashes and often contain pow-erful chemicals. Many of the same reactions that can occur when taking a pharmaceutical drug can occur with these herbal reme-dies, but at least we know the major risks before we take a drug; we know what we are getting when we swallow the pill and we have a good medical reason for taking the drug. Why risk a possible dan-gerous reaction from an herbal supplement that is not being care-fully monitored for contaminants and content?

To tell you that herbs are useless would not be the truth. There is plenty of research on chemicals that have been extracted from herbs and some of this research is very promising. Researchers are extracting chemicals from different herbs that are anti-inflam-matory, anti-cancer, anti-thrombotic, and free radical squelching. Chemical extracts from some of these herbs may prove to help out some of the symptoms of disease. But that does not mean I would trust just any company to get the right herbal extract in the cor-rect amount into a pill that I would take, or, heaven forbid, give to my child. One study evaluated over-the-counter herbal remedies and tested them for the ingredients stated on the package. Only 50% percent had the amount of herb stated on the package; oth-ers had ranges of herb that varied by over 20%. One of the brands tested did not have any evidence of the herb found in the product!

Now, I must tell you that I am a believer in *vitamin and min-eral supplements!* I recommend that most of my patients take a supplement, but I do not believe that supplements will cure any disease. Since many people do not get the daily amounts of vita-mins and minerals that are required for maximal body function-ing, the supplement can help to replace essential minerals and vit-amins in amounts that may be hard for some people to ingest on a daily basis. Calcium and vitamin D supplements are a perfect example of this. Calcium is a mineral that is required for good bone health. It is found mainly in milk products, but can also be found in some vegetables such as kale and broccoli, and even in nuts such as almonds. If a diet is not rich in these foods, it is likely that not enough calcium is being ingested. This is where a good supplement is helpful.

The situation with vitamin D is even more complicated. The body makes vitamin D in the skin when exposed to sunlight, but is dependent on the amount and absorption of sunlight exposure. Dark skinned individuals and people living in northern climates tend to make less vitamin D and require more from dietary ingestion. The problem is that vitamin D is not found in a wide variety of foods with the main food sources for Vitamin D found in fortified cereals, milk and fish. A vitamin supplement is very helpful for many people. A very important point about vitamin supplements is the labeling. All vitamin and mineral supplements list the exact amount of vitamins and minerals that you are swallowing in the pill. Many herbal supplements do not tell you how much plant is in the supplement; even more troubling is that they *cannot* tell you what chemically active substances are in the supplement.

It is time to answer the question about herbal supplements with respect to cold and flu prevention. I need to be very careful because I do not want to point a finger at any one particular manufacturer of herbal supplements. I am letting the public know that many of the manufacturers of herbal supplements make unsubstantiated and misleading claims about cold and flu prevention. These products make billions of dollars despite a lack of medical evidence to support their claims. Why is this happening? The misinformation chain is at play here.

Most viral illnesses are self limited and disappear after a few days. Taking an herbal supplement during an illness may make it seem as if the supplement sped up the recovery. Taking the supplement at the "first sign" of an illness can be misleading as well. There are some people who think they are getting a cold if they sneeze. They take their magic supplement and don't get the "cold" they weren't going to get anyway. Then they tell a friend about this "great" supplement who then tells two friends, and so on.

Along with marketing and brand recognition, a product is suddenly making millions for some company that has no scientific data to back up any claims that the product is effective. At the present time, science says there is no cure for the cold. The only thing that can protect someone 100% from getting a cold is not getting exposed to the virus.

I will now look at the evidence for and against the efficacy of common herbal ingredients found in natural remedies that claim to prevent or cure colds and flu, and come up with evidence-based information on the use of herbal supplements for viral illnesses. I will focus on the most widely used ingredients found in some popular supplements.

Herbal supplements commonly contain a combination of Lonicera, Forsythia, Schizonepeta, Ginger, Chinese Vitex, Isatis Root, and Echinacea. Let's take a look at each herb individually and see what we come up with in terms of fighting off colds and flu.

First is Lonicera, a honeysuckle plant used in many herbal supplements. One study was able to extract 12 chemicals from the plant and found them to have anti-oxidant capacity as well as anti-inflammatory effects. Specifically, the researchers were able to show chemicals from this plant inhibit the enzymes cycloxygenase 1 and 2, which are the same mechanism that drugs like Voltaren and Naprosyn use to exert their anti-inflammatory effect. Finding out that some of the chemicals in this plant are beneficial to humans is no surprise. Many medications used in western medicine have been extracted from plants, about 30 percent. As I said before there are many benefits to plant phytonutrients, but I also said that many plants have toxic chemicals that can be very dangerous to humans if ingested. The public should not be taking in unknown amounts of plants in a dehydrated form. As far as the data on Lonicera fighting off colds and flu... there is no data

Next on the list is Forsythia, a flowering plant. At this time this is a plant that should be in our garden, not in pills. Researchers have isolated two chemicals in the plant that exhibit strong anti-inflammatory activity and anti-bacterial activity. The isolation of the compounds from this plant that exhibit anti-bacterial activity can have profound effects on medicine if harvested properly.

Bacteria are ever changing and able to destroy many of the antibiotics we use to kill them, therefore limiting their usefulness. It is always important to find new ways to defend against bacterial infection and the finding of antibacterial chemicals in Forsythia may be very promising for future use. Again, I did not find any data to support the use of this flowering plant in supplement form to help prevent colds and flu.

Schizonepeta is third on the list and is an herb grown mainly in China. Essential oils isolated from this plant were found to be a good insecticide! This means the plant has natural pesticides, and as I stated in a previous chapter, natural pesticides are as carcinogenic in rodents as manmade pesticides. It is therefore possible to extrapolate this information and state that remedies with schizonepeta oils may be carcinogenic. This information needs to be taken very seriously because, as you can see, all that is natural is not benign. Again there was no data to substantiate its use to fend off colds and flu.

Ginger is a well-known plant. It is a very useful plant in the same family as cardamom and turmeric. The plant root is safe when eaten and has been used for centuries in cooking. The best data on the usefulness of ginger extract is its usefulness as an anti-nausea agent. It appears to be safe and effective in alleviating pregnancy-induced nausea and post-operative nausea. The dose of the plant needed to have the anti-nausea effect is 1 gram per day. Ginger also has anti-inflammatory effects and I highly recommend using it when cooking. I also recommend some ginger products, like ginger tea, when I am treating an acute gastrointestinal virus in my patients. The data on alleviating nausea is very real. However, there is no data to substantiate any claim that it can prevent viral infections.

Another herb used in supplements that claims cold and flu prevention is Chinese vitex. Extracts have been shown to have estrogenic properties and research is looking into using the extracts as hormone replacement therapy. The extract also acts on opiate receptors and is effective in preventing PMS. There is still much more research that needs to be done before this herbal extract can ever be considered for use to help women with menstrual or menopausal symptoms, and none of the research pointed toward warding off colds and flu.

Isatis root used in some supplements has some good data to show anti-bacterial properties but not anti viral properties. The extract from this plant, when made into an eye drop formulation, has been shown to have excellent efficacy in treating bacterial conjunctivitis. Again, we have the possible makings of a new antibiotic but no data to show its usefulness against viral infections.

Last on the list is Echinacea which is made up of nine different plant species and is one of the most common nutraceuticals ingested. Current research has evaluated the use of Echinacea for the common cold. There are over 200 viruses that can cause the common cold. A meta analysis looked at fourteen studies on this herb and concluded that the use of Echinacea not only shortened the duration of the cold, but also decreased the risk of getting a cold. Echinacea, when used preventatively, can reduce the incidence of a viral cold by 68%. However, it only reduces the incidence of Rhinovirus, the most common cold virus, by 35%. Researchers are not sure how Echinacea works to stimulate the immune system, but it appears to up-regulate various factors that put the immune system into action. There are many different chemicals found in the plant, and they vary in concentration depending on what part of the plant is used to make the supplement. The plants contain flavonoids and other phytonutrients, but it is not known if one chemical alone or the combination of chemicals causes the preventative effect with cold viruses.

So there you have it. Only one herb out of the most commonly used for cold and flu prevention remedies has any possible effect on cold viruses. The public needs to realize that these herbal remedies are real pharmaceutical agents that act in a very similar way as common medications. The natural herbal extracts can kill bacteria, mimic estrogen, alleviate pain, kill bug larvae, or decrease inflammation, but they can't prevent or treat the flu virus. All of these reactions may be happening in your body when you take some of these supplements.

Herbal remedies should be treated the same as all other drugs in the United States. They should be regulated by the FDA with a watchful eye on the products, contaminants and use of these potentially potent plant extracts. I can't recommend the use of these extracts, mainly because we don't know what we are getting when a pill is swallowed. The research that I reviewed generally evaluated purified extracts of chemicals from the plants. The exception to this was the study done on Echinacea, but the dosage shown to have the antiviral effect was three times higher than the amount found in many common herbal cold remedies.

It would be great to take a pill that makes us live longer, gives us more energy, prevents cancers, alleviates hormonal symptoms, buffs up our immune system, or improves our memory, but that pill does not yet exist. The important point I am making is that every person who takes herbal supplements needs to know how the plant extracts are manufactured, where the plants come from, what other ingredients are in the supplements, and how impurities are removed. Adults who take other medication should make sure the chemicals from the supplements do not interact with their drug regimen.

As a pediatrician, I can't recommend combination herbal remedies for children because of the risk of contamination with metals, lack of standardized dosing, risk of reactions, unknown effects of the herbs, and the possibility that what is stated on the package is not what is being ingested.

It is interesting to find out that some of these plants have very potent anti-bacterial activity. Many of the staunch advocates of herbal remedies seem to also be adversaries of modern medicine, especially of antibiotics. It seems that modern medicinal agents and ancient herbal remedies are all very similar both in chemical composition and action in the body. But because herbal remedies come in a "natural" form, people assume they are better, safer, and can do no harm! Think again.

17

What Can I Do to Help Fight Off Germs?

There are some people who can be exposed to numerous illnesses but never get sick. There are other people who are what I call a "walking culture medium"—any virus that blows their way sets up house in their body. The reason that some people seem to fight off every microbial challenge is imprinted in the DNA that regulates the many facets of their immune system. It is the same reason why other people are more prone to illness. That is not to say that genetics is the only player in how well we fend off bugs. There are other major variables that affect our immune system, and these are the variables we will talk about. What can we do to keep our immune system functioning at peak level?

The immune system allows us to live in this world filled with the living organisms that continually bombard our system. If the immune system is weakened or defective, we would not be able to defend ourselves against the dangers of eating fresh foods, since the bacteria that sit on fresh foods would pose a threat to the weakened host. The molds that are found in our basements, bathrooms, foods, gardens, and virtually everywhere in our environment, would turn from innocuous annoying microbes to an invading army that could kill. A small cut in the skin could become a festering, oozing boil, and walking through a crowded mall or subway would be like swimming in a swamp. Without the immune system to immediately gobble uninvited microbial agents, our lives would be in danger with every breath.

All parts of the immune system must be in working order to defend ourselves against invasion of foreign microbes. Our skin acts as a coating to protect invaders, the hairs lining our nose and respiratory tract are used to "sweep out" organisms, our stomach acid can kill much of the bacteria that we ingest each day, and cells that line all parts of our mucous membranes and intestinal system are ready to destroy invaders. This is called our innate immune system; our skin and "innards" that are lined with cells, mucous, and enzymes to pillage a non-invited microbe. If an organism gets past our initial line of defense, we have plenty of more cells to help us out. This helpful system is our adaptive immune system. It includes antibodies and different types of white blood cells that are designed to destroy microbes or any molecule that is foreign to the human body. Some white blood cells (WBC) make antibodies specific to the invading bug (I use the term bug to describe any virus, bacteria, fungi etc. that does not belong in our body) while there are other WBCs that will "eat" any invading microbe. Most offending bugs can be fought off by a healthy immune system before they kill us. Unfortunately, there are some new super bugs (like Ebola virus or avian flu) that are mutating our way, and even the healthiest immune system can't fight them off (that is a whole different chapter).

How well we defend against the constant bombardment of unwanted microbes depends on many different factors. I am going to talk about the most recent data on the modifiable factors that contribute to fending off infectious illnesses.

The most obvious habits that will keep the immune system in tip-top shape is to stay well nourished, get enough sleep, and exercise regularly. Some less known immune modulating factors include stress, certain amino acids, laughter, probiotics, prebiotics, aging, certain nutrients, sleep apnea, meditation, and keeping a healthy colon.

I love talking about nutrition, so let's start with how we can "nourish" our immune system. Because every vitamin is needed for our immune system to function at peak level, it is important to make sure we are getting the proper amounts of vitamins in our diet each day. The antioxidant vitamins and minerals like vitamin C, E, selenium, copper, and zinc counteract damage from free radicals and help to modulate the immune system. Vitamin B6, B12, folate, and iron all help support the immune system, and vitamins A and D play a role in cellular immunity as well as antibody production.

Vitamin A is one of the more important vitamins for immune health. As I said before, it not only helps antibodies function well but also helps the cells that direct the immune traffic. We are much more likely to have an illness turn deadly if vitamin A levels are low. Measles virus is a dangerous virus, but when vitamin A intake is low, as is commonly seen in underdeveloped countries, measles becomes a major threat to life, especially for children. Vitamin A is found in abundance in yellow and orange vegetables and to a lesser extent in green vegetables. Sweet potatoes and carrots contain the most vitamin A by a landslide. It is important to note that it is much better to get the vitamin through foods rather than taking a supplement with large amounts of vitamin A. Large amounts of this vitamin can be toxic. So avoid supplements with megadoses of vitamins.

Vitamin C is another powerhouse for our immune system. Vitamin C's role in the immune system is very diverse. It is an anti-oxidant to squelch damaging free radicals, it increases natural killer cells in our body that destroy viruses and bacteria, it increases white blood cell movement, and it also increases the production of a subset of immune fighting cells. Vitamin C levels decline rapidly when our bodies are stressed, so it is very important to keep up vitamin C levels when we are ill. The role of vitamin C and infections has been studied for decades; the biggest question about vitamin C is whether it helps to fight off the common cold. There are some people who subscribe to the belief that taking large doses of vitamin C is a good way to fend off a cold. These are the people who take mega doses of the vitamin at the first sign of illness. Vitamin C in large doses is relatively benign and does not cause toxic reactions like mega doses of vitamin A or iron, but it can cause diarrhea and upset stomach. Whether it works or not is a different story. The latest large study clarifies some questions but still leaves room for more research to be done.

Vitamin C, when taken every day, or *preventatively*, does appear to help shorten the duration of colds in adults by 8% and in children by 13%—not very impressive numbers. However, in people who are experiencing short-term physical stress (most of us probably feel we fit into this category) the use of preventative vitamin C decreased the incidence of colds by 50%—an impressive number. Fortunately, many of us don't fit into the category of those experiencing short-term physical stressors; the stressors that were identified in the study were military personnel in sub-arctic temperatures, marathon runners, and skiers. This leaves the majority of us in the category of preventative vitamin C having a minimal effect on the duration of a cold. Unfortunately, the effect was dose dependant with very high doses showing the minimal improvement.

Almost all fruits contain some amount of vitamin C, but common fruits that are packed with vitamin C include kiwi, guava, grapefruit, orange, mango, and papaya. I advise parents to make fruit smoothies when kids are sick to help continue their nourishment since many children reduce their food consumption during illnesses. Refreshing fruit drinks not only help with hydration; they can deliver a power packed nutrient punch. Buying frozen fruits is a good way to make sure you have some of the more exotic fruits on hand year round, while still ensuring that the nutrients are present in the fruits.

The bottom line appears to be that taking large preventative doses of vitamin C is not beneficial to the general population, although it is beneficial under extreme physical stress and cold. I may increase my vitamin C intake the next time I go on a ski trip, but for now I will keep eating my fruits and vegetables and take a regular multivitamin.

My mother always told me to wear my hat and gloves when I went outside, and who was I to go against the advice of my mother; after all she did know everything (at one time in my life). Many generations have believed that getting a chill would increase one's risk for getting a cold. As it turns out there are many "old wives tales" that end up having some truth to them. How would they have survived being passed on for generations if there wasn't an inkling of truth to them? For example, the old adage about eating chicken soup to cure a cold has indeed proven to be helpful in fighting off illness. In the past I came across research to help prove the theory that standing near an open window with a wet head would increase the risk of getting a cold. One study theorized that becoming chilled caused a change in the ph of the nasal mucous, making it easier for viruses to invade the respiratory cells.

This sounded very reasonable to me, so for many years I have defended my mother and all mothers who insisted that their children dress warmly when going out into the cold. The problem is that newer research does not back up the idea that getting a chill will increase your risk for illness. I have a hard time believing this, especially after reading the research on vitamin C. The use of vitamin C in preventing colds was best under physically stressful circumstances, two of them in cold weather. I believe that our increased susceptibility to illness when exposed to cold occurs when the body is stressed by trying to keep warm. The body expends energy at a higher rate when subjected to cold temperatures. If the body is being stressed by cold temperatures AND at the same time a virus blows your way, the body has most of its energy diverted to the task of keeping warm and may be less able to fight off an invading organism. Illness does not just happen from being cold. It takes a bug to do the damage, and if the bug happens along while your body is struggling to keep warm, the physiologic stress may just be enough to let a virus set up shop in your nose.

Zinc is next on my list. Zinc is an essential mineral for the body to be used by 100 different enzyme systems and is essential for proper immune function.

One of the more interesting aspects of zinc nutrition is that with adequate intake, it is a very potent immune stimulant; likewise, when levels of zinc intake are inadequate, the immune system does not function well. In fact, zinc is so important to proper immune function that one of the top ten causes of morbidity and mortality in developing countries is zinc deficiency. On the other side of the coin, taking excess amounts of zinc causes immune suppression! This is a very important point because there are very few healthy people in developed countries walking around with a zinc deficiency. Despite this, many people take zinc supplements that are advertised to help fight off colds when they feel the start of a cold. It is possible that it may end up doing more harm than good by suppressing immune function.

The final word on zinc supplementation and cold symptoms is not yet complete. The most recent study on zinc supplementation taken at the onset of a cold did in fact show a reduction in the duration of the cold symptoms from seven days down to four days in the supplemented group. The supplement had to be taken every two to three hours! Most of us (me included) are unable to take a pill more than two times a day, let alone every two to three hours.

It is much better to get zinc from foods than from supplements. Foods that are good sources of zinc include beef, turkey, pumpkin seeds, wheat germ, lentils, sunflower seeds, beans, chicken, and oysters, which come in at number one for zinc content. Zinc absorption is inhibited by foods high in phytates (found in legumes, whole grains), so high protein meals are better suited for good zinc absorption.

Many of us are all too familiar with the scenario of feeling over-whelmed with work. Whether it is the over-scheduled parent running from event to event or the business woman working 10 hour days, we know that stress takes a toll on a person. Stress affects our mental state, but it also has a tremendous effect on our internal cellular functioning. Although the external signs of stress like weight loss or gain are obvious, the internal signs are not readily evident. What we don't see is the tremendous effect on our internal cellular functioning. The brain has the power to affect all things in humans. How well infection is fought off is one of them. When the body is stressed mentally or physically, the hypothalamic pituitary axis becomes over stimulated (remember the fight or flight response we learned about in school?). The result is a myriad of hormonal changes which affect how well the immune system can fight off a microbial insult. I am sure many of you reading this book can remember an illness that followed a stressful event.

Each year in my practice I usually see an influx of patients complaining about not feeling well just before the end of the school year. They complain of headaches, tiredness, colds, or just "not feeling good." The vast majority of the time it is the stress of finals at the end of the year that causes their immune system to be suppressed; the end result is an increased risk of catching every virus that blows their way. Unfortunately, stress is hard to avoid. It would be nice if we were in control of all physical stressors that come our way. But we can, to a certain degree, control our mental stress. The state of mind we choose to walk around with, either the "stressed out" or "let it roll" state of mind, has an effect on immune function. Constant worrying, depression, and distress decrease immune function, whereas optimism, good coping skills, laughter, and a good support system will help to counteract the depressing effects that stress has on the immune system. The mental choices we make have an effect on whether we catch more of the illnesses that we are exposed to or whether we can fight them off.

Let's talk about another one of my favorite topics: exercise. There is a long list identifying the many benefits of exercise, but who would have thought that it can help to fight off infection. It has been shown that people who exercise moderately have increased mucosal antibodies, which are infection-fighting molecules lining the nose, lungs, mouth, and intestine to fend off the bugs that blow our way. This means that exercising between 3–30 minutes per day at LESS than 75% of cardiovascular capacity can help fend off illnesses.

I have long known that exercise has an effect on all bodily functions, but I also always felt that when I exercised I was MORE likely to get ill. This is contradictory to what I just said. Well, believe it or not, medical science has backed up what I have always felt and I am sure what many of you avid exercisers out there already know. The exercise issue is not a simple one when it comes to immune function. Those of you who choose to work out more intensely, such as doing 60 minutes of exercise at greater than 75% cardiovascular capacity not only have a decreased mucosal antibody response, but also have a decrease in the number of killer cells. This would mean that individuals who exercise at greater intensity levels will more likely get sick IF exposed to bugs after their workout. Therefore, it appears that the level of the intensity of the exercise is a factor that regulates the amount of antibodies lining our respiratory and gastrointestinal mucosa that is our first line of defense against infections. So exercise regularly, but don't overdo it or your immune system will suffer.

One of the most abundant amino acids (protein building blocks) in the body is glutamine. Glutamine is a non-essential amino acid which means the body can manufacture glutamine. Immune cells as well as the cells lining the GI tract use glutamine as fuel. Glutamine is made in the body and increases white blood cell functioning. It is the preferred fuel for the GI tract and helps to keep the cells lining the tract healthy. If the body is depleted of glutamine, the GI tract function to act as a barrier to invading organisms is impaired. Interestingly, when we exercise, the demand for glutamine increases and the muscle glutamine becomes depleted if not replaced. Arginine is another amino acid that affects the immune system by stimulating the growth of the immune cells. Our body can make glutamine and arginine, but when substrate runs low the body can be in trouble. Foods that contain glutamine are high protein foods such as chicken, turkey, and fish, whereas peanuts, tree nuts, seeds, and soy are all high in arginine.

The next big topic on improving the immune system is the use of probiotics. There are now many foods advertised to contain "healthy bacteria" to promote health. But are we to believe these claims and eat food with ADDED microbes? If the added bacteria do help us, how do we know if the bacteria are still alive when we eat the food. Does it even matter? How much do we have to eat to have a positive health impact? Is it possible that probiotics could cause sickness? There are a lot of questions to answer, so let's get started.

We must understand what a probiotic is before we can answer these questions. A probiotic is a microbe that has some beneficial effect on the host. It would seem odd that eating live organisms can be helpful to us when I am discussing how aggressively our immune system works to get rid of foreign microbes. The key word is "foreign;" the microbes I am talking about in this section will enhance our "natural microbial flora." Our natural microbial flora consists of the 100 trillion bacteria that reside inside our intestine to help maintain healthy intestinal cells. These microbes are essential for maintaining a normal intestinal barrier; they help stimulate antibody production, create mucous to protect the lining of the intestine, and create antimicrobial substances that help to fight infection. The flora is also important for digestion, absorption, vitamin synthesis, and energy production. The health of our colon plays a very big part in our overall health, and what we eat plays a big part in our colon heath.

Does eating microbes in the form of probiotics help humans? There are many proven benefits of using probiotics. Some of these include decreasing diarrhea associated with antibiotic use, improving colonic cell integrity, decreasing the duration of intestinal infections, and positively affecting immune function by enhancing the immune response to invading foreign microorganisms. Some strains have even been shown to decrease the severity of symptoms of respiratory infections. One of the most important aspects of keeping healthy is maintaining colonic (intestinal) cell health. We need to feed our gut, and believe it or not, eating certain bacteria is one of the ways to improve our ability to fight off unwanted bacteria and viruses.

It appears that certain strains of microbes affect our health in different ways. The most popular and safest families appear to be lactobacillus and bifidobacterium. Not all strains have the same beneficial effect on the host; the benefits are *strain* specific. For example, if the label of a food says it contains live cultures of lactobacillus and does not give the exact strain, such as lactobacillus reuteri ATCC 55630, we can't assume it is the strain to help fight off colds. The strains that have been most identified as having a positive effect on the immune system are bifidobacterium lactis HN019, bifidobacterium lactis Bb-12, and lactobacillus casei DN114001.

The amount of a probiotic that is needed to have a beneficial effect is not known. Most studies use numbers that start in the 1 billion colony-forming unit range, but because there are no standardized amounts, I can't comment on the best dose to use. Probiotics need to be eaten every day to have the positive benefits mentioned above. Another issue of ingesting probiotics in foods includes how the manufacturer maintains a live colony count. There are no regulations that check the amount of probiotic in foods. There are independent consumer groups that do research on different food products to check on the live colony count after purchase. However, even if the probiotic microorganism is dead, it still may have a beneficial effect.

The use of prebiotics is on the rise. Prebiotics are different from probiotics in that prebiotics can be used as food for the more beneficial bacteria in the colon. Prebiotics do not have a direct effect on the immune system, but they can directly affect the colonic milieu in a positive way, and thereby help us to boost our immune system. Common prebiotics are the fructans that are naturally occurring oligosaccharides found in onions, bananas, artichokes, garlic, and asparagus. Another fructan that may sound familiar is inulin, a chicory fructan, which is added to foods to increase nondigestible food content. The non-fructan prebiotics are the resistant starches found in raw potatoes and unripe fruit. Many aspects of good health come down to eating fresh fruits and vegetables in abundance.

We can do many things to stimulate our immune system. There are also many avenues that cause a depression in immune function. Fasting decreases immune function, as do high-fat diets, sleep deprivation, obesity, prolonged intense exercise, and excessive alcohol consumption.

When it comes to helping our body fight off germs we need to exercise in moderation, get enough sleep, laugh a lot, decrease mental stress, meditate, eats lots of fruits, vegetables, nuts, and legumes, stick to poultry and fish as the main sources of protein, and start to eat more live bacteria in the form of probiotics.

Section V

Cell Phones and New Problems

Every day there is some report released about items that we commonly use that may potentially harm us. These sensational stories are often reported to the public before enough studies have categorically declared something to be truly harmful. This is done for other reasons than to simply inform the public. After all, controversy makes headlines! However, some widely publicized topics have indeed helped the public. One of the topics I am talking about is the recent obesity epidemic in children, which has been fervently addressed in the media and is finally coming to a plateau. Others include the endless cell phone and radiation controversy, and the recent identification of certain chemicals used to make plastics that may pose a health threat.

The obesity epidemic has spurred many people to try to help curb the problem; I am one of them. I wrote a book and made an exercise DVD for children and parents called "Growing up Healthy" to attempt to teach parents ways to ensure their child does not become a statistic in this epidemic. Unfortunately, there are many other people who are trying to help, but do not have any medical, nutritional or pediatric training. I want to inform people about a new trend of ideas written about by non-medical people attempting to help parents, but who instead may cause more harm than good.

The use of microwave ovens and cell phones generated a lot of chatter when they first became popular. It seems that the microwave chatter has disappeared, but the cell phone chatter (no pun intended) has amplified. I will present information on electromagnetic radiation and cell phone usage, particularly in our children.

There has also been some frightening information circulated on the Internet and in the media about plastic materials. These and other questions are going to be answered in the following chapters.

18

The Obesity Epidemic: How to Avoid Becoming Part of the Statistics

The obesity problem that is occurring worldwide is taking a huge toll on adults and an even bigger toll on our children. One of the most important ways to promote a good diet and ensure good health is to include fruits and vegetables in our daily meals. But many adults do not get the recommended amount of fruits and vegetables on a daily basis, and children fare even worse. If adults aren't eating their fruits and vegetables, who is going to teach the children to eat good foods?

This is the heart of a big problem occurring in the world today. It takes a lot of energy to make sure your child eats well and even more energy if you are not a good eater yourself. In our harried society it is very easy to turn to fast foods and quick-processed meals. If eating well is not a priority, fast food can become a way of life. The ones who suffer the most from a perpetual avoidance of healthy foods like fruits and vegetables are our children. They have been born into a world where drive-through restaurants are a billion dollar business. They do not have the advantage that most adults and many parents have because they were children before the fast food industry was at its peak. This meant that most of us had no choice except to eat what our parents put on the table. In the past more mothers were stay-at-home moms who cooked meals that were better balanced than today's typical family meal. So at the very least we were likely to have grown up with a more healthy diet as children, until we went astray as adults in the processed high-sugar and high-fat food world. The current estimate is that 60% of adults are overweight, and as a society we are getting heavier and heavier. Our children will not stand a chance of a healthy future if we do not change this course.

We are seeing health initiatives all over the place, from Bill Clinton to Nickelodeon. The government, television, school systems and big industry are all trying to get the message out to eat healthier foods. Much of this is because of the obesity epidemic occurring in children as a result of not eating a healthy diet from a young age.

As society tries to come up with solutions to help children eat well, the most recent trend are cookbooks that teach parents how to disguise healthy foods as the usual kid fanfare. Parents are finding this to be an easy way to attempt to get their children to like food that is good for them. Unfortunately, the most likely result of this technique will be a more unhealthy generation of children!

Let me explain. Growing up is a time when habits are developed and basic life survival mechanisms are learned. One of the most important habits that a child can learn is to eat fruits and vegetables and to have a healthy lifestyle. The combination of eating well with regular exercise can prevent 60% of disease related deaths as they age.

If children are not taught how to eat properly, they will grow up without the understanding that eating well can perpetuate good health. Getting children to eat brownies with hidden legumes, or sneaking vegetables into a macaroni and cheese dinner, does not reinforce good food habits. Instead, it sends the message that macaroni and cheese and brownies are foods that can be eaten regularly. The end result will be children who never learn which food is good for them who become adults with poor eating habits. This will result in your child becoming an adult who is at much greater risk for diseases. The World Health Organization has estimated that over 20% of heart disease, 15% of GI cancers and 11% of strokes are related to poor vegetable intake.

All children need to be taught how to eat well; it does not come naturally to most kids. This requires that parents talk about the benefits of eating vegetables and fruits. It is not a good idea to disguise foods to try to fool your children. The idea is to teach your children and to lead by example. It is never a good idea to deceive your children.

The effort it takes to make healthy meals, to be a good role model, and to teach your children how to eat well, is nothing to sneeze at. Parents need to understand how important it is to make this effort. The easy way out is to give in to your children and not bother to teach them about the importance of good eating habits. The easy way out is to disguise foods so that you don't have to hear the whining when the vegetables come out. But the easy way out will ultimately cause more harm than good.

Do not disguise healthy foods in order to present them to children. If you want to make mashed potatoes with cauliflower, fine, as long as you tell your child what is in the food and why it is healthy. Be a teacher to your child.

19

Cell Phones: Are They Safe?

A big part of my job includes time on the phone handling a myriad of different topics throughout the day. I like to wear headphones when I talk on the phone because it allows me to move around my office while I am talking, as well as being much easier on my neck muscles. One day while I was on the headset speaking with a patient, a loud, vibrating noise started to come through the headset; it sounded as if a plane was going to land in my office! The first time it happened I was quit startled and stood up trying to figure out where the sound was coming from. The sound eventually stopped and I did not think twice about it. But it happened another time, and again the sound startled me. This time I realized that my cell phone in my pocketbook on the floor was ringing. I realized that this horrific sound from my headset was caused by the radio waves coming into my cell phone that the headset was picking up as a signal. I was able to physically "sense" the radio waves coming into my cell phone because I not only heard them, but I even felt them from the vibrations of the headphones. It was startling to think that my cell phone was generating waves with such power, that they caused the loud, vibrating sound picked up by my headset. I have since learned that cell phones emit only low frequency non-ionizing radiation. This is contrary to my first thoughts of my "audio" encounter. However, low frequency radiation does not translate into harmless radio waves.

Let's talk more about the electromagnetic field and radio waves before we go into deciding if cell phone usage is safe. The electromagnetic spectrum comprises a large waveband of radiation defined by frequency and wavelength. Short wavelengths have higher frequencies and emit lots of energy that can cause damage to human DNA. An example of high frequency short waves are gamma radiation and x-rays. Long wavelengths have lower frequencies and emit small amounts of energy; examples of these include radio waves and microwaves.

Understanding the electromagnetic spectrum gives us insight into the radiation we are exposed to each day. The highest energy radiation in the form of gamma radiation is ionizing radiation or DNA-altering radiation. There are many uses of gamma radiation. From CT scans, nuclear medicine scanners, and even cancer treatment, gamma ray energy is harvested for beneficial uses. The next strongest form of ionizing radiation are X-rays; no further elucidation is needed on the beneficial use of x-rays.

Ultraviolet radiation is next on the spectrum of energy that is ionizing radiation. The UV spectrum includes UV A, UV B, and UV C rays. The UV A radiation reaches the earth and does its damage by producing free radicals in the skin, increasing the risk for skin cancers. UV B radiation is partially absorbed by the ozone layer and can cause significant skin damage. UV C rays are completely absorbed by the ozone layer, however, with the gradual depletion of this layer more of the damaging form of radiation can reach the earth. The spectrum moves on to non-ionizing radiation (non DNA damaging) in the form of visible light, infrared radiation, microwaves, and radio waves.

As you can see, we are exposed to electromagnetic radiation in various forms each and every day—from stereos, radios, the sun, microwave ovens, electrical appliances, wi-fi networks, power lines, wiring in buildings, as well as from cell phones.

For most people cell phones are no longer a luxury but are, instead, a necessity. It is hard to imagine leaving the house without your cell phone. The days of instant communication are here and are going to stay. Gone are the days when my pager would go off, and I had to pull over to use a pay phone to return a phone call. With instant technology my answering service can call my cell phone no matter where I am and can connect me to a patient's phone within seconds. It would be very difficult, if not impossible, for many to give up the advantages mobile communication technology has given to the world.

But what if it was causing an increased risk in tumor formation or causing damage to our DNA? If mobile technology was causing serious damage to humans *over a short time span,* we most likely would have seen it already. We know that cell phone use does not seem to be causing cancer or brain tumors *over the very short period of time that they have been in use.* The big problem is whether use of cell phones can increase the risk for tumors, cancers, and other problems over a longer period of time. This is especially important when it comes to young children who are using cell phones at young ages and will be using them for 70–80 years or more.

Cell phones work by transmitting and receiving radio waves. The following is a basic explanation of what happens when someone makes a call on a cell phone: The cell phone emits radio waves that are received by a radio base station in the nearby area. Radio base stations are set up all over the world and consist of a tower or antenna set up on top of a building. The radio waves are sent out parallel to the ground so very little radio energy reaches the ground from these stations. The signal is then sent to another base station which receives it and sends it on until it reaches the receiver of the call. When a call comes into your cell phone the radio waves come into the antenna of the phone wherever it may be— in your pocket, purse or belt. (This is an important point that I will come back to shortly). Realize that this is an extremely simplified explanation, but I think the basic idea is clear.

The International Commission on Non-Ionizing Radiation Protection has set the limits for the amount of electromagnetic radiation exposure that is considered "safe." (What is considered safe amounts of radiation exposure in one person may not be safe for another person; genetics may play a big part in how people respond to these radio waves.) It is the *responsibility* of governmental and local agencies to check radiation levels around power lines and mobile phone stations to make sure radiation emission is at a safe level. Each cell phone also has a specific absorption rate (SAR) which is the amount of energy that is emitted from the phone that becomes absorbed by the body. The FCC (Federal Communications Commission) regulates the maximal allowable SAR level. Cell phone companies must make sure that the SAR level is below the level set by the FCC before it can put the phone on the market. There are a lot of layers of regulation that the government needs to monitor to make sure that we are safe from excess radio frequency emissions.

The Internet contains a plethora of misinformation on many different topics. A recurring theme in my book is to remind people to read everything with a critical eye and to beware of people with an agenda. Information is coming from many places in the media, and articles are being written every day reviewing possible dangers of cell phone usage. So far, however, the FDA says phone use has not been "scientifically linked" to any adverse health outcomes. A good number of the studies I reviewed say something to the contrary. They showed cellular effects from the radio waves emitted from cell phones. Cellular effects can possibly amount to a myriad of problems. Why is it necessary to wait for damage to human health before things change? More importantly, why do we take the risk of damage to our children before we make changes to standards and recommendations for cell phone use safety.

I want to share some of the reported effects of cell phone usage and then look at the real data and evaluate whether these claims are real or hype.

Reported problems from cell phone usage included immune system suppression, cancers, brain chemistry effects, DNA damage, headaches, Alzheimer's disease, sleep disorders, and even autism.

Brain tumors and cell phone usage have been the most talked about since early use of these devices. As I said before if there were a *significant short term* connection, we would have seen it already; this is not to say that the long term users will not be at risk. Looking at the accusation of a relation between cell phones and cancers, I came across many good studies that refuted the

link between brain tumors and cell phone usage over the relatively short time they have been around and widely used. But the final
word on tumors and cell phone use is not out yet. A large review
recently looked at the incidence of brain tumors and cell phone
use. The study could *not* conclusively say that cell phones were
causing an increase in a certain type of brain tumor called a
glioma, however, they could not say that cell phone radiation was
not causing the increase. The study did show an increase in
gliomas on the same side of the head that cell phones were used
and concluded that more research needs to be done. Another
recent meta-analysis did not reveal any association between cell
phone use and brain tumors.

My worry is for our children who will use cell phones over their
complete lifetime. The radio wave radiation that is emitted from
phones has a greater effect on young children than it has on
adults. There are two main reasons for this. First, the younger
skulls of children absorb more radio wave radiation than the
skulls of adults; it therefore penetrates deeper into the brain. This
is because the exposure radiation being emitted from the cell
phone is closer to the whole body resonance frequency in children. Every part of the human body has what is termed a "resonance frequency." This is the frequency of radiation that excites
the molecules in the body. Visualize this by imagining a tuning
fork. When the tuning fork is hit, it starts to vibrate and continues
to vibrate after it is hit. The radiation absorption stimulates the
molecules in the body to vibrate, which may cause harm. More
absorption of radiation into the body can only translate into more
cellular damage, and the area of radiation absorption is in the
brain. The second reason children have more radiation damage is
due to the rapidly growing cells in their bodies. Children are in a
very active growing state with more cell division and growth than
in adults. This poses more potential for damage to occur from
radiation.

The next possibility is that cell phones cause DNA damage
which can subsequently cause cancer. This accusation may be a
major issue for users over long periods of time if it turns out radio
waves from cell phones cause DNA damage. This could mean

increases in many different types of cancers over the next 50–100 years. Any time DNA damage occurs, whether it is in the form of breaks, replication problems, or repair problems, the risk for unchecked cell replication can occur.

A study looking at cell phone radio frequency radiation on human white blood cells in the lab did not show any damage done to the DNA after 24 hours of continuous exposure to SAR values simulating the energy that would occur by cell phone use. Another study simulated the radiation exposure that occurs from mobile phone base stations on human cells. The cells were exposed to continuous radio waves for six weeks and were than evaluated for neoplastic cell transformation. The researchers reported no cell transformation occurred. One study did find that DNA rewinding (remember DNA is in a double helix formation) was affected by radio waves, but the ultimate outcome of altered DNA rewinding was not stated in the study.

The results of these studies are important, however, since reports show that 40–55% of radio wave energy emitted from the cell phones is absorbed into the skull, while even more radiation gets absorbed into a child's skull. Researchers need to look more closely at the brain cells and the response to radio waves. The results of a study that looked at the effects of short-term radio wave phone emissions on different types of brain cells revealed that mechanisms that stimulate cell death are turned on by radio wave radiation. All cells in our body have a protective mechanism to self destruct. This self-destruction cascade is the system that is turned on by radiation. This means that when we use our cell phones, we are increasing our *chances* of destroying brain cells; the study does not conclusively translate into an absolute loss of brain cells, but indicates an increase in the activity in the DNA that is used to shut the cell down. This means brain cells may be dying from cell phone use—a worrisome situation when we think that our children are absorbing more of the radiation and possibly losing brain cells!

Cell phone radiation appears to change protein expression in some cells. All cells use and make proteins to function properly. Any alteration in the structure, production, or function of any protein can have profound effects on the body. For example, if the proteins that are used to transport glucose into the cells are changed in any way, the end result could be devastating. The degree of alteration of the protein expression depends on the cell type. There have been good studies that included different types of brain cells in order to document an effect of radio waves on the alteration of protein expression. It appears that radio waves affect protein production in certain brain cells more than others. The endpoint of the alteration in protein expression is not known and needs to be studied in more detail.

To sum it up, there does not appear to be any direct carcinogenic affect on DNA from cell phone radio waves. However, the radio waves do have an effect on the expression of proteins in the cell that is guided by DNA programming, as well as also having an effect on the brain cell's death regulation mechanisms. Radio waves do have effects on cell functions, and at the present time we do not know if this translates into future cancer or not.

The accusation that cell phone radio emissions cause Alzheimer's is an interesting one. Even with so much research on Alzheimer's disease, none of it has accused the use of cell phone radio waves as a cause of the disease. We do know that there is an accumulation of beta amyloid protein in the brain of afflicted individuals and that this toxic protein is produced by the action of enzymes that are proteins. If radio waves affect the production of this particular protein enzyme system, it could very well be associated with an increased risk of Alzheimer's. Another possible link might be found in the increase in cell death mechanisms and radio waves because the end point of Alzheimer's disease pathology is brain cell death. For now we cannot make any conclusive link between Alzheimer's and cell phones.

When making a claim that something has an association with autism, it is of particular importance to make certain that the data to back up the accusation exists. To make an unfounded claim is not only irresponsible but may give false hope to the parents of autistic children that amounts to nothing short of cruelty. It is known that developing fetal tissue is very sensitive to environmental toxins. Electromagnetic radiation may prove to have many effects on the adult human with none of them being of any health significance. However, it might be entirely different for the developing human fetus.

There is very little data about any association between cell phone use and autism. It appears to be mostly speculation. The rise in the rate of autism seems to coincide with the widespread use of cell phones, but making a temporal association has very limited validity. Cell phone radiation does affect cellular protein production. For the developing fetus any alteration in protein production could have dramatic effects. The alteration of a few cells early in fetal development could affect a whole system, including the brain. Nothing is proven, but it seems prudent for pregnant women to use land-line phones more frequently, not to carry the cell phone on a belt around the belly and decrease overall cell phone use while pregnant.

The immune system allows us to live in this world filled with microbes. If the immune system is weakened or defective, we would not be able to defend against the microscopic dangers that lurk everywhere. The effects of radio waves on the blood components of the immune system have been evaluated in some studies. Overall, it appears that routine use of cell phones does not have any significant effect on the immune system.

Whether cell phone usage causes headache, increased blood pressure, or behavioral changes is still under study. If talking on a cell phone gives you a headache or you feel it changes your personality ... hang up. So far nothing conclusive has come out about blood pressure changes related to cell phone use, but I would not be surprised if cell phone use is linked to increased blood pressure.

An observational study done in 2008, however, revealed a possible link between cell phones and sperm count. It appears that radio frequency radiation affects sperm counts and decreases sperm motility. The sperm counts are not decreased to below what is considered normal, but it does, nonetheless, appear to decrease the overall number of sperm. This may have to do with the heat generated from cell phones. Sperm production occurs in the testicles, which are outside the body for good reason—the temperature is lower and is better for sperm production. Men tend to carry cell phones in their pockets near their genitals. The phone produces heat that may subsequently raise the testicular temperature. The other consideration is that the radio waves have direct effects on the sperm. It is logical to recommend that men should keep their cell phone out of their front pockets.

Society has become more and more dependent on cell phone usage. We should be wary of this new technology and the increasing electromagnetic radiation that comes along with it, especially when it comes to children and pregnant women. I think it is a good idea for adults to use the phones sparingly.

As for the effect on children, we should proceed with caution. The data is telling us that children are more at risk for problems resulting from radio wave radiation than adults. It is even possible that the fetus is at risk. Children are going to be exposed to more radio wave radiation over time than their parents and grandparents. They are also going to have absorbed more radiation into their bodies over their lifetime. The long term effects of this are yet to be seen and I am seriously concerned with the possibilities. We are continually exposed to more and more of this type of energy, and we are seeing more cases of autism, childhood cancers, brain tumors and behavioral issues including, ADHD. Is there a correlation? No one knows the answer to this question. My recommendation is for children to use a commercially made antenna guard that reduces radio wave emission and to urge that cell phone use be restricted (this is good for many other reasons as well). The trend is to use text messaging which brings the radiation from the phone away from the brain (and the cell phone bill way up). Because there are still more questions than answers, pregnant women should try to use land-line phones and avoid any possible extra electromagnetic radiation.

With all that being said, I will not stop using my cell phone anytime soon, but I will continue to use it sparingly. As for children, cell phones should be viewed as an unknown variable for their future health.

20

Are Plastics Safe Containers for Food and Beverages?

There has been some scary information circulated around the Internet about plastic materials and the leaching of dangerous chemicals into our food and drinks. Is it safe to drink bottled water? Is it safe to give your baby milk in his bottle each day? Will freezing or heating the bottles give off a toxin that may kill us someday?

The newest scare on the chemical front is our exposure to the chemical bisphenol A, also known as BPA. BPA was first made in the lab in 1891, but it was not researched until the 1930s when chemists were researching estrogen-like compounds. BPA was found to mimic the effects of estrogen, but chemists found that DES was a stronger estrogen-like compound, so BPA was put aside for future use. BPA was shelved until the 1950s when its use increased as a building block to make polycarbonate plastics and epoxy resins. The polycarbonate plastic is a hard, clear, heat-resistant plastic with good electrical resistance that is virtually shatterproof. It is used in many products, such as electronics, automobiles, CDs, DVDs, food containers, baby bottles, water bottles, dental sealants, juice and milk containers, and many more items. The epoxy resin is used as a protective coating in metal cans, paints, and adhesives. Over 90% of people tested in the United States by the Center for Disease Control have been found to have BPA residue in their urine. This means that almost all humans have been exposed to this chemical, and since the half-life of BPA is short, it means that we are exposed to this chemical on a regular basis.

The question is about how we are exposed and what is happening to humans as a result of this exposure. The hard tough plastic that is made with BPA is used for many household purposes, but the problem with BPA is that it is not a stable chemical and the bonds holding the chemical in place start to break down over time. The result of these unstable bonds is that BPA has the potential to leach into the food and drink that are housed in polycarbonate plastics. New plastic, as well as old, used, scratched-up plastic, has the potential to let out BPA.

Studies have shown that BPA is leached from cans that are lined with polycarbonate resin and storage containers that are made with polycarbonate plastic. Studies have found that BPA leaches from baby bottles and can be detected at 1–3 parts per billion. Water bottles made of polycarbonate plastic have been found to leach BPA at levels of 0.1–4 parts per billion. Plastic tableware was shown to leach BPA at levels of less than 5 parts per billion. BPA has been found in baby formula that was housed in BPA containing cans as well as in many other canned foods. The higher the fat content of the food, the more likely BPA will be leached from the lining of the cans and end up contaminating the food or drink. There are other ways we are exposed to BPA besides food and drink housed in polycarbonates. We are also exposed to BPA through environmental contamination of water which occurs from leakage from landfills. The thought of water that humans drink each day being contaminated from landfill leakage is extremely disturbing!

Hard, plastic, sport, water bottles have been touted as better for the environment because they are reusable and will not fill up landfills as quickly as the softer plastic bottles that are disposed of after one use. These hard plastic bottles do, however, contain BPA and therefore may pose a risk to humans.

We need to ask and answer more questions before we have enough information to decide if we should be avoiding BPA-containing products. The next important question that needs to be answered is how much BPA do humans ingest, and what is a safe level?

It is estimated that humans ingest BPA between 0.00048 mg/kg/day to 0.0016 mg/kg/day based on blood and urine levels. The most disturbing part of this is that children were found to have the highest intake of BPA based on their urine and serum levels. The reference dose established by the U.S. Environmental Protection Agency is 0.05 mg/kg/day. A reference dose is set as a standard that is the maximal exposure amount that is deemed to be safe for humans. With a reference dose set at 0.05 mg/kg/day and the average range of intake much, much lower than this dose, it would *seem* that we are safe from harm from this chemical. Unfortunately, the story does not end here. The reference dose, set years ago by the EPA, is based on old research. Since then many new studies done on lab animals have shown that BPA intake at levels *lower* than the reference range can cause harm.

I mentioned that BPA has the ability to imitate estrogen. Because it is a hormone-like chemical, BPA is a known endocrine disruptor. The outcome of exposure to endocrine disruptions in a developing animal includes gene malfunctioning, reproductive pathology, brain changes, and many other physiologic changes. These physiologic alterations occur as a result of the gene malfunctioning, which has a cascading effect on many developmental pathways. This can result in long-term disability or even death.

So what does this all mean? To sum up the information so far, we know that BPA is used to make hard polycarbonate plastics used in hundreds of products. It is an estrogen mimic, an endocrine disrupter and almost every human ingests BPA on a regular basis as it leaches out of polycarbonate plastics and landfills. The next step is to determine what levels of exposure cause harmful effects.

The reference dose set by the EPA is *higher* than levels that have been shown to cause harm in many animal studies. As stated before, the studies that looked at BPA levels in humans found that children had the highest levels; this means they have the greatest continual exposure. As is often the case, studies done on lab animals found that the most damage happened when BPA exposure occurred in the developing or newborn animal.

The more recent studies on BPA exposure are very alarming. One study found BPA levels to be three times higher in women who had recently miscarried as compared to controls. They also found evidence of chromosomal abnormalities in the miscarried fetuses. BPA exposure in lab animals has been shown to increase risk for breast and prostate cancer, reduce sperm count, impair immune function, cause genital malformation, and cause behavioral changes that include hyperactivity and impaired learning. These studies used BPA in amounts lower than the EPA reference dose.

Tied into BPA exposure is a common question of the cause of early puberty in girls. Everyone blames it on the "hormones" in food. This has not been proven. What has been proven, however, are the problems that BPA can cause when pregnant women are exposed. Studies have shown that fetuses of pregnant women who ingested BPA had higher blood levels of BPA than the mother. This means that BPA is concentrated in the fetuses! A study in pregnant mice fed very low doses of BPA (much lower than the EPA acceptable intake) found their offspring to move into puberty earlier. The ramifications of children going into puberty early are multifaceted; puberty and BPA exposure does not end with the cause and effect study I just mentioned. A possible indirect effect of exposure can occur as well. Fetal exposure to estrogen-like compounds has been linked to obesity. The endocrine disruption from the exposure of a fetus to BPA causes an increase of the likelihood of obesity; children that are obese are more likely to go into puberty at an earlier age. It is obvious that we need to be doing more research on all possible exposures to chemicals by fetuses and children. The search may lead to the answers we have been searching for as to causes of clusters of children going through early puberty.

Dissecting the information on this topic was not an easy task. A well-done study noted an industry bias when it comes to BPA research. The researchers reviewed over 100 studies that were conducted to find possible effects of BPA exposure. It was found that studies done by "industry" consistently found no detrimental effects that could be attributed to BPA. However, 90% of the studies that were funded by the government or academic institutions *did* reveal problems with BPA exposure. Does this tell us that it is difficult to trust studies when they are funded by groups that stand to gain or lose money as a result of the final outcome of the research? There is a dichotomy among industrial agencies and academic researchers on the opinion of BPA exposure and the possibility of health risks. Are the industry-funded studies skewed? I would like to think that this is not the case. One explanation could be that new techniques in research have come a long way in the past few years. The ability to detect chemicals down to parts per trillion as well as the ability to detect miniscule changes that occur in a cell as a result of chemical exposure can make some studies done in the past 20 years outdated. If most of the industrial studies are older studies, this could explain the discrepancy in results. It still remains that new studies are coming out that are identifying the risks of BPA exposure, but for now, the FDA and other agencies contend that it is "safe." However, more research needs to be done.

The Bottom Line

As far as answering the question, "Is it safe to drink water from plastic bottles?" the answer is, "It depends." It depends on what type of plastic the container is made from, and who is eating or drinking the contents.

The hard, clear, polycarbonate plastics are the ones that contain BPA. BPA, even in small doses, is an estrogen mimic and endocrine disruptor. The effects this may have on a developing human are too much to risk. I would recommend that pregnant women avoid exposure to this chemical as much as possible. There is data to show that BPA is found in baby formula housed in cans lined with epoxy resins that have BPA. Some of these formulas are used every day by thousands of my patients. I am very troubled by the studies I read about BPA and endocrine disruption, especially in relation to the damage that can occur when fetuses are exposed to this chemical. I can say that I do see a good number of baby girls who develop breast tissue in the first few years of life. The breast tissue usually resolves uneventfully after careful observation by the pediatrician to make sure there are no other signs of puberty. Pediatric text books advise the physician to look for any possible exposure to estrogens, and if there are no other signs of puberty to observe the child closely until the breast tissue resolves. Can it be that this entity described in text books as a self-limited, benign condition is instead due to intermittent BPA exposure in the young babies? It makes perfect sense to me! I have seen girls develop breast tissue on and off more than once before they finally went into puberty, and now I have another possible reason as to why this happens. I even saw a young, healthy, baby boy for a one year physical who I noted to have breast tissue development. This is NOT a benign condition, and I immediately did a full evaluation on the baby. He was drinking large amounts of soy formula at the time. After all the blood work came back normal and I followed the baby closely, the only conclusion that I could come up with was that the phytoestrogens in the soy formula were the cause of his breast tissue development. He was switched to cow's milk, and eventually the breast tissue resolved. I am now convinced that this baby boy was somehow being exposed to BPA. Because I switched him from the canned formula his breast tissue resolved (thank goodness).

Once my patients enter into puberty after their early breast development (possibly from BPA), I cannot say that they are safe from issues developing in the future long after I have taken care of them. Since BPA is not a banned substance, at this time formula companies are allowed to use the epoxy resins to line their cans of baby formula (there are some companies that do not use BPA in their cans).

The soft, plastic, water bottles that are used for one-time use do not contain BPA. An important issue is to question why people drink water from a plastic bottle that will cause more pollution, release toxic dioxin into the air, and use up landfill space. Why not drink tap water that is more regulated than bottled water and does not require the use of plastics? If you want portable water, use steel containers. They are reusable and do not break down like plastics do.

It seems clear that all of us need to avoid BPA exposure. It even seems that BPA use should be severely restricted, if not banned, since it can cause harm to the developing human. Think of the catastrophic effects that the endocrine disruptor DES had on the babies that were exposed to DES as a fetus. We should not have to learn that certain chemicals cause harm by waiting until people are severely harmed by them.

The Bottom Line

I have discussed many different topics in this book, some of which are very controversial. Some of the topics could not be addressed completely because of ongoing research that has not given definitive answers to the problems posed. I presented the information, and if the information was not conclusive, I gave my *opinion* on the topic.

Talking about the topic of vaccines and autism always peaks the interest of people; after all, almost everyone is either a parent, grandparent, brother, sister, aunt or uncle, and is concerned about the well-being of children. Many people, after finding out that I am a pediatrician, ask me about vaccines and autism. I always tell them the same thing: there is no connection between autism and vaccines and there never was a connection. An irresponsible article started a whole chain of events that have been difficult to turn around. When I relay this information to people, they almost universally come up with the same question: "If the vaccines are not the cause of the increasing autism rate, then what is causing the increase in autism?" The answer that I give these inquiring folks is "I am not sure." If they want to hear my opinion, I tell them that the changing diagnostic criteria include many more children than were previously included, and children are being diagnosed at a younger age, both of which increase the incidence rates. There is a lot more to the story of autism than just those two areas that I did touch on in the book, but much more research has to be done to definitively answer that question.

It would be complete speculation to say that pesticide exposure in early pregnancy may have something to do with the increasing incidence of autism, but I am one mother who is going to make sure my girls do everything that is possible to avoid pesticide exposure before and during pregnancy.

The BPA problem is not going away any time soon, mainly because of the big money industry that relies on this chemical for profits. The best advice I can give to people is not to worry if they are exposed to it in small quantities because the body can handle small doses of this endocrine disruptor without causing permanent harm. But it is paramount to understand that the fetus cannot handle this chemical and any exposure could be disastrous! My recommendation for women who are planning to get pregnant or are already pregnant is to drink liquids from glass and to avoid canned foods. BPA is found in landfills, so there are no guarantees that this will eliminate BPA exposure completely, but it is a good start.

The bottom line is that this is not going to be the end of the story for many of these controversies. I am, however, quite sure that vaccines and thimerosal do not cause autism. I am sure that sugar in the quantities we consume is dangerous for humans. I am sure that the form of sugar that modern society uses most (high fructose corn syrup) is contributing greatly to morbidity in the world. I am sure that vaccinating your child is crucial to maintaining a standard of health that we can all enjoy in the 21st century. I am sure that there aren't any hormones in cow's milk that are causing problems in children. I am sure that both before and during pregnancy the avoidance of recreational drug use, mercury-laden fish, alcohol, and smoking, as well as being fully vaccinated, will improve the chances of having a healthy baby. Finally, I am sure that eating a well-balanced diet with fresh fruits and vegetables, having a full set of vaccinations, exercising the mind and body regularly, having cranberry, apple, pomegranate or grape juice throughout the week, drinking a glass of red wine with dinner, limiting red meats, seeing a medical doctor regularly, and reducing physical and mental stress, will help us move closer to finding the fountain of youth.

Afterword

I hope I have helped people to gain a better understanding of the many medical issues currently reported on in the media. I read the most active and recent research on these topics and used my medical expertise to answer the questions that were posed.

My desire is to spread true medical information. Too many non-medical people are becoming involved in giving medical information to the public. Unfortunately, this is causing more harm than good. The population should not be listening to politicians and activists who use medical issues to gain power by appealing to people's emotions about controversial topics such as autism or vaccines. The public should not be getting medical advice from actors, vitamin companies, magazines, or non-medical experts in other fields.

People need to turn to their doctors if they want to get medical advice. If they heard a disturbing report on television, they should call their doctor for clarification on the topic. I am happy to answer questions my patients pose to me each day. If I am not familiar with the topic or problem, I will do research to find out the information. A doctor's understanding of the disease process is necessary when analyzing research studies. It is also helpful in determining whether the study was well done or not. All too often, studies are published that are poorly done.

I realize there are many people who have formed firm opinions about many of the topics I touched on, and will be reluctant to change their minds. But I want everyone to be aware of the REAL medical information, not the information that they read on the Internet or hear from a friend.

I recently had a mother come to my office with her son for a routine physical. The mother informed me that her son had allergies and he was suffering from congestion, itchy nose and eyes. The young boy had been prescribed an FDA approved antihistamine that I have been using for years on my patients without any adverse events. The mother did not want to use the recommended medicine. Instead she wanted to use something "more natural." She showed me the product that she was using, which contained quercetin and two other herbal ingredients. I asked the mother why she thought that this herbal product was not a medicine and why she was willing to use it on her son. I explained to her that the allergy product recommended to her was a pure product and any possible side effects were known. I reminded her that the herbal supplement was medicine, but unknown medicine.

She did not agree with me. She kept insisting that the supplement was "more natural." Again, I explained to her that this supplement had at least three different chemicals (probably much more than that), and we could not even be sure of the ingredients. She did not want to listen to me when I tried to educate her and to help her son. She refused to understand that she was not only using more medication than she had to, but she also could not be certain what medication she was giving to her child. Instead, she told me she had a naturalist that she uses and I would "never convince her" that herbs can be dangerous and contain many chemicals—because after all, they do come from nature. That was a frustrating visit!

The political arena is getting involved with medical issues; many of us don't trust politicians to do an honest job when it comes to our money, so why would we think they know what they are talking about when it comes to medicine? The issue of thimerasol in vaccines was touched upon at the beginning of the book. I explained how there is no evidence to support any link to its use and autism. The action to remove thimerasol from vaccines was based on the data from the more toxic methlymercury, but, with that being said, it is still better that it has been removed from most U.S. vaccines. I am bringing this up because I recently have had two encounters with politicians who were discussing vaccines, but clearly had no medical knowledge as they spread misinformation.

One of these encounters involved a talk show with a politician and an autism activist. The politician had been helpful in a proposal ensuring that all children under 18-years-old and all pregnant women receive thimerasol-free vaccines. But the politician went on a verbal rampage stating that his constituents that were diagnosed with autism were all told by their pediatricians that they would "outgrow" the delay. I politely waited until I could inform him that pediatricians are heavily trained in childhood development. It is an important part of the board exam that pediatricians must take before they can say they are board certified. I also told him that I don't know of any pediatricians who, when confronted with a child who was not developing normally, would say that he or she will "outgrow" the delay. Why was this politician stirring up so much anti-pediatrician sentiment?

The autism activist then went so far as to use the words "big cover-up" when talking about thimerasol. A COVER-UP! People such as these make up their own stories or use inflammatory words to spread their propaganda for their own agendas and appear as if they could care less about the truth. Why would the thousands of pediatricians in the United States take a vow to care for children, but then give shots that we "know" could cause problems like autism or mercury toxicity? The answer is that pediatricians spend their days and nights caring for the children of the world and would never knowingly put a child at risk. Because we spend our days giving out vaccines, the pediatrician is usually the first one to see a side effect from a shot. Pediatricians know that these vaccines and the ingredients used as preservatives to help make the vaccines safe have never caused autism. If there was any association between disease and vaccines, pediatricians would not continue to give the vaccine to children.

It has been my pleasure to take care of children, and I look forward to many more years doing what I love. It is my hope that when you have a question that pertains to medicine, you will seek out the answer from someone who has the medical qualifications to answer the question.

Suggested Readings

Moschandreas, D.J., and S. Karuchit et al. "Exposure Apportionment: Ranking Food Items by Their Contribution to Dietary Exposure." *Journal of Exposure Analysis and Environmental Epidemiology,* 12(4) (July 2002): 233–43.

Groth, Edward III, Ph.D., Charles M. Benbrook, Ph.D., and Karen Lutz, MS. "Do You Know What You're Eating?: An Analysis of U.S. Government Data on Pesticide Residues In Foods." February, 1999 *Consumers Union of United States, Inc. Public Service Projects Department Technical Division.*

Das, R., A. Steege, S. Baron, J. Beckman, and R. Harrison. "Pesticide-related Illness Among Migrant Farm Workers in the United States." *International Journal of Occupational and Environmental Health* (2001) 7:303–312.

Huffling, Katie, BSN. "The Effects of Environmental Contaminants in Food on Women's Health." *Journal of Midwifery & Women's Health* 51(1) (2006): 19–25.

Beier, R.C., and H.N. Nigg. "Toxicology of Naturally Occurring Chemicals in Food." *Foodborne Disease Handbook,* Vol 3 (Hui YH, Gotham JR, Murrell KD, Cliver DO, eds). New York: Marcel Dekker Inc., 1994, 1–186.

Gold, L.S., T.H. Slone, B.N. Ames, and N.B. Manley. "Pesticide Residues in Food and Cancer Risk: A Critical Analysis." *Handbook of Pesticide Toxicology,* Second Edition (R. Krieger, ed.), San Diego, CA: Academic Press, 2001, 799–843.

Magnuson B.A., G.A. Burdock, J. Doull, R.M. Kroes, G.M. Marsh, M.W. Pariza, P.S. Spencer, W.J. Waddell, R. Walker, and G.M. Williams.

"Aspartame: a Safety Evaluation Based on Current Use Levels, Regulations, and Toxicological and Epidemiological Studies." *Critical Reviews in Toxicology.* (2007) 37(8):629–727.

Finn, J.P., and Lord, G.H. "Neurotoxicity Studies on Sucralose and Its Hydrolysis Products with Special Reference to Histopathologic and Ultrastructural Changes." *Food and Chemical Toxicology* (2000) 38 Suppl 2:S7–17.

Roberts, Eric M., Paul B. English, Judith K. Grether, Gayle C. Windham, Lucia Somberg and Craig Wolff. "Maternal Residence Near Agricultural Pesticide Applications and Autism Spectrum Disorders Among Children in the California Central Valley." *Environ Health Perspectives* (2007) 115(10):1482–1489.

vom Saal, Frederick S., and Claude Hughes. "An Extensive New Literature Concerning Low-Dose Effects of Bisphenol A Shows the Need for a New Risk Assessment." *Environmental Health Perspectives* Volume 113, Number 8, August 2005.

Calafat, A.M, X. Ye, L.Y. Wong, J.A. Reidy, and L.L. Needham. 2007. Exposure of the US population to bisphenol A and 4-tertiary-octylphenol: 2003–2004.

vom Saal, FS, S.M. Belcher, L.J. Guillette, R Hauser, J.P. Myers, G.S. Prins, W.V. Welshons, and J.J. Heindel et al. 2007. Chapel Hill. "Bisphenol A Expert Panel Consensus Statement: Integration of Mechanisms, Effects in Animals and Potential Impact to Human Health at Current Exposure Levels." *Reproductive Toxicology* 24:131–138.

Christensen, H.C., J. Schuz, M. Kosteljanetz et al. "Cellular Telephones and Risk for Brain Tumors: A Population-based, Incident Case-control Study." *Neurology* (2005) 64: pp 1189–1195.

Thompson, W.W., Price, C., Goodson B. et al. for the Vaccine Safety Datalink Team: "Early Thimerosal Exposure and Neuropsychological Outcomes at 7 to 10 Years." *New England Journal of Medicine.* 2007; 357:1281–1292.

Wintergerst, E.S., S. Maggini, and D.H. Hornig. "Contribution of Selected Vitamins and Trace Elements to Immune Function." *Annals of Nutrition and Metabolism.* 2007; 51(4):301–23.

Fleshner, Monika. "Physical Activity and Stress Resistance: Sympathetic Nervous System Adaptations Prevent Stress-Induced Immuno-suppression." *Exercise and Sport Sciences Reviews* 2005; 33(3): 120–126.

Zhao, T.Y., S.P. Zou, and P.E. Knapp. "Exposure to Cell Phone Radiation Up-regulates Apoptosis Genes in Primary Cultures of Neurons and Astrocytes." *Neuroscience Letters.* 2007; 412(1):34–8.

Nylund, R., and D. Leszczynski. "Mobile Phone Radiation Causes Changes in Gene and Protein Expression in Human Endothelial Cell Lines and the Response Seems to be Genome- and Proteome-dependent." *Proteomics.* 2006; 6(17):4769–80.

Dai, Qi MD, Ph.D, and Amy R. Borenstein, Ph.D. et al. "Fruit and Vegetable Juices and Alzheimer's Disease: The Kame Project." *The American Journal of Medicine* Volume 119, Issue 9 (September 2006).

La Rue, A. "Nutritional Status and Cognitive Functioning in a Normally Aging Sample: a 6-y Reassessment." *American Journal of Clinical Nutrition,* January 1997; 65(1): 20–9.

Tokar, M., and B. Klimek. "Isolation and Identification of Biologically Active Compounds from Forsythia Viridissima Flowers." *Acta Pol Pharm.* 2004; 61(3):191–7.

Spangler, R., K.M. Wittkowski, N.L. Goddard, N.M. Avena, B.G. Hoebel, and S.F. Leibowitz. "Opiate-like Effects of Sugar on Gene Expression in Reward Areas of the Rat Brain." *Molecular Brain Research.* 2004; 124(2):134–42

Takeuchi, T., O. Tsutsumi, Y. Ikezuki, Y. Takai, and Y. Taketani. 2004. "Positive Relationship Between Androgen and the Endocrine Disruptor, Bisphenol A, in Normal Women and Women with Ovarian Dysfunction." *Endocrine Journal.* 2004; 51:165–9.

Index